U0251714

ATLAS OF LOWER LIP RECONSTRUCTION
下唇再造术图谱

（德）余健民　著　　Author：Yu Jianmin
余健民　绘图　　Painting：Yu Jianmin
（余健民医学博士、口腔医学博士　Dr.med.Dr.med.dent.Yu Jianmin)

192年来96种下唇再造术回顾

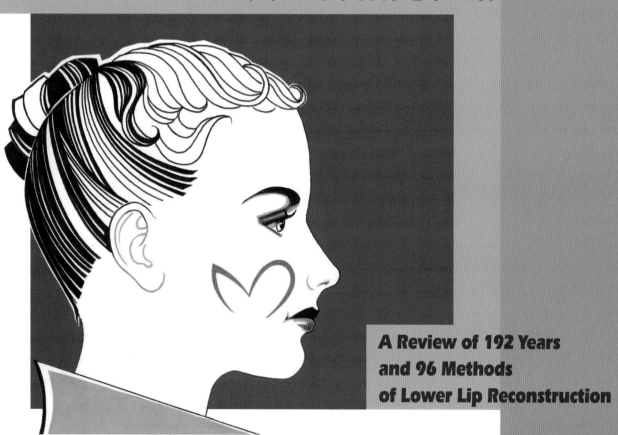

A Review of 192 Years
and 96 Methods
of Lower Lip Reconstruction

北方联合出版传媒（集团）股份有限公司
辽宁科学技术出版社
沈阳

图书在版编目（CIP）数据

下唇再造术图谱 /（德）余健民著. —沈阳：辽宁科学技术出版社，2017.1

ISBN 978-7-5381-9949-9

Ⅰ．①下⋯　Ⅱ.①余⋯　Ⅲ.①唇—整形外科手术—图谱　Ⅳ.①R782.2-64

中国版本图书馆CIP数据核字（2016）第227895号

出版发行：辽宁科学技术出版社
　　　　　（地址：沈阳市和平区十一纬路25号　邮编：110003）
印 刷 者：辽宁新华印务有限公司
经 销 者：各地新华书店
幅面尺寸：210mm×285mm
印　　张：10.5
插　　页：4
字　　数：220千字
出版时间：2017年1月第1版
印刷时间：2017年1月第1次印刷
策 划 人：倪晨涵
责任编辑：陈　刚　苏　阳
封面设计：余健民　张　珩
责任校对：徐　跃

书　　号：ISBN 978-7-5381-9949-9
定　　价：128.00元

投稿热线：024-23280336
邮购热线：024-23284502
E-mail:cyclonechen@126.com
http://www.lnkj.com.cn

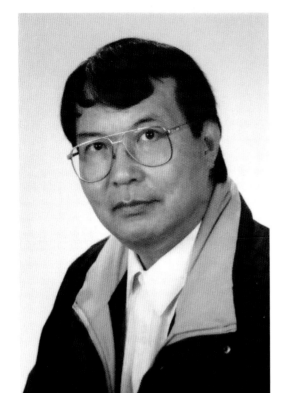

作者简介

　　余健民，1969年毕业于中国医科大学，之后从事临床工作，学习口腔医学和在中国医科大学做口腔颌面外科医生工作，有时画手术和解剖图。1980年因亲自设计、解剖和制备手腕标本并绘制由中国医科大学编写的《实用解剖图谱》而获得中国国家奖，深受美国、德国、瑞士、奥地利等国著名专家的赞扬。

　　1982年后在德国弗里德里希－亚历山大－埃朗根－纽伦堡大学口腔颌面外科医院从事科研、教学和医疗工作。1995年获得医学博士学位证书和口腔医学博士学位证书，这两篇博士论文均获得最优秀成绩，又获得医生执业证书、口腔医生执业证书、口腔颌面外科专科医生证书和整形手术证书。他的诊所被当地评为五星级诊所。

　　1988年和Steinhaeuser教授、Janson教授编绘《颌骨矫正外科学》。独创"余氏下颌关节脱位复位法"和"余氏下唇再造术"。发表多篇医学论文。

　　自幼受父亲和叔叔艺术熏染，后师从大师周铁衡、霍安荣先生，在医疗工作之余，进行美术和书法创作，在德国不同城市举办了七次书画展。很多国家总统、国王、总理等收藏余健民为他们画的肖像画。1986年余健民获德国奥地利艺术家奖。

Yu Jianmin, graduated from Chinese Medical University in 1969, then worked as a doctor and sometimes drew for Medical Operations and Anatomy, studied Stomatology and worked as an Oral and Maxillofacial Surgeon in China Medical University. In 1980, he won the national prize for personal design, dissection and preparation of hand and wrist specimen and drawing *Practical Anatomy Atlas* compiled by China Medical University, for which he gained great appraisal from famous professors coming from the USA, Germany, Swiss and Austria, etc.

From 1982, Dr. Yu began to take up research, teaching and medical treatment in Oral and Maxillofacial Surgery Hospital of University of Erlangen-Nuremberg (in German: Friedrich-Alexander-Universität Erlangen-Nuernberg)in Germany. Until 1995, he had been honored with MD degree and MD degree in Stomatology. His two doctoral dissertations were both top graded. At the same time, he had been awarded Doctor's Practical Certificate, Oral Doctor's Practical Certificate, Certificate of Oral and Maxillofacial Surgeon and Certificate of Plastic Surgery. His clinic is rated as Five-Star clinic by patient.

Dr. Yu Jianmin compiled and drew *Maxilloorthopedic Surgery* together with Prof. Steinhaeuser and Prof. Janson in 1988. Original therapy: "Yu's replacement of mandibular joint dislocation" and "Yu's lower lip reconstruction". And Dr. Yu has published many medical research articles.

Being influenced by his father and uncle for art from the childhood, later study with the masters Mr. Zhou Tieheng and Mr. Huo Anrong, Dr. Yu often makes painting and calligraphy creation after medical work. He had held Painting and Calligraphy Exhibition for 7 times separately in different cities of Germany. Many presidents, kings and prime ministers over the world collect portraitures that Dr. Yu created for them. Dr. Yu Jianmin ever won German-Austrian Artist Award in 1986.

序言（1）

　　本书是关于下唇由于病变施术后造成缺损进行修复再造术的参考工具书。通过文字和插图描述了从1823年开始的DELPECH技术到今天一共192年的时间段里95种不同的技术后，余健民博士提出并研发了自己新的、可运用于下唇缺损2/3情况下的下唇修复技术。书中，余博士详细介绍了所有的手术方法，促进了口腔颌面外科在下唇修复再造领域的进一步发展，并对由于病变或创伤造成下唇缺失需要进行修复的患者有所帮助。

　　1980年余博士由于绘制了《实用解剖图谱》上下肢部分的插图获得了中国国家奖。余博士凭借其精湛的绘画艺术能力，用208幅精准的插图，完成了对下唇修复再造技术的论述和总结，并最终编辑成册。本书对于未来口腔颌面外科和整形手术的学习提供了巨大的帮助。1989年他的文章《肿瘤切除术后下唇再造新方法》发表于医学专业期刊《European Journal of Plastic Surgery》，此后获得了欧洲众多同行对此方法的优越性、重要性和创新性的认可。

　　当时德国弗里德里希–亚历山大–埃朗根–纽伦堡大学口腔颌面外科医院、口腔颌面外科门诊医院院长Dr.E.Steinhäuser教授评价余博士，首先是一名医生和口腔颌面外科领域的专家，在拥有无与伦比的医术同时，还是一位艺术家。此外，医院里的所有医生都能从余博士的实践知识中获益。他的艺术家天赋是对其医术的完美补充。余博士也是一位具有高贵品质的同事，这一点得到了他所在医院上司、助手以及患者的充分肯定。本书特别是对于年轻的同行提供了大量的参考。它的完整性大大方便了下唇修复再造术选择完美方法的检索。

　　本书使用两种文字编写，即中文和英文。由此对于医学学生，包括一般外科、整形外科以及口腔颌面外科学生学习不同语言在专业术语上的表达提供有价值的参考。与该书同时出版的还有余先生的《面颈部美容外科手术彩色图谱》，余博士的这本著作在其专业领域中有无与伦比的价值，同时对于新一代的同行同样有着巨大的帮助。

滕卫平　教授

原中国医科大学校长（2000年9月—2003年9月）

2014年5月26日

This book is a compendium for the reconstruction of the lower lip after defect resection. After description and illustration of 95 methods of lower lip reconstruction from around the world that have begun with the technique according to DELPECH in 1823 and therefore cover a period of 192 years, Dr. Dr. Yu Jianmin made a breakthrough with a new method of reconstructing a new lower lip with a defect of two thirds. All operation methods were vividly illustrated by Mr. Yu. This gave impetus to further development of oral and maxillofacial surgery in the area of lower lip reconstruction which could help patients to obtain a new lower lip that was lost through illness or trauma.

In 1980 Mr. Yu was awarded the National Award of China for his drawn figures in the *Atlas of Practical Anatomy* that is dedicated to the upper and lower limbs. He used his superb painting skills to make a summary of the methods with 208 highly precise and masterly figures that became a picture compendium of lower lip reconstruction. This book provides a great convenience for future study of oral and maxillofacial as well as plastic surgeries. In 1989, his article titled, *A New Method for Reconstruction of the Lower Lip after Tumor Resection* was published in the medical magazine *European Journal of Plastic Surgery*. After publication of this article, many European peers thought that this method is outstanding, prominent and innovative.

The former director of the Clinic and Polyclinic of Oral and Maxillofacial Surgery at the Friedrich-Alexander-University Erlangen-Nuremberg Professor Dr. Dr. E. Steinhäuser wrote in his evaluation that Mr. Yu has an extraordinary talent as a physician and artist and that he is an excellent doctor and specialist for maxillofacial surgery. Furthermore, all doctors of the clinic can benefit from his surgical knowledge. His artistic gift is an ideal addition to his medical competence. Mr. Yu is an extremely valuable colleague who is tremendously appreciated by his superiors and co-workers as well as his patients. This book is a particularly valuable reference for younger colleagues. It can facilitate researching the perfect method for lower lip reconstruction, thanks to its completeness.

This book is illustrated in two languages: Chinese and English. It is a valuable reference for medical students as well as general, plastic, oral and maxillofacial surgeons to study medical terms of the respective languages. With this book, Mr. Yu publishes another *A Color Atlas of Aesthetic Surgery of the Face and Neck*. His work has made an unmatched contribution to this field and will be a great benefit to future generations.

Professor Teng Weiping

Former President of the Medical University of China

Date of Term: September 2000 until September 2003

May, 26th 2014

本书由余健民博士撰写。余博士曾学习和工作于沈阳的中国医科大学。该校以解剖学著称，并拥有研发中国皮瓣的优秀师资队伍。作为一名学生，余博士能够从这样的经历中获益，并在完成学业后开始各类撰写、绘画工作。

他是一位拥有丰富颌面解剖知识，且才华横溢的外科医生。除了这些卓越的手术技巧，他也是一位艺术家，能够创作出色的解剖图。他渊博的人类解剖学知识、出色的手术经验和艺术技巧都被融汇到了这本下唇再造书中。

除外伤，唇癌是下唇不足的主要原因之一。通过这种外科手术达到良好审美和功能恢复是高质量生活的必要前提。

余博士给出了192年来96种下唇再造术回顾。在介绍中，显示口周区域的解剖结构。在给出唇部再造的外科手术，即通过直接缝合、推进皮瓣、旋转皮瓣、远位皮瓣之后，余博士提出了他的下唇再造方法，对外科手术给出了很多有价值的建议，并通过精湛的绘画描述方法表达出他的外科手术过程。

此书以可理解和明确的方式编写为中文和英文，阅读时简单快捷。为了能更好地便于理解，手术操作的途径和过程用大量优秀绘图来说明。总之，本书为每一位处理再造手术的医生，尤其是为下唇再造建立了一个非常有价值的标准。

总而言之，本书为我们的医生提供了不可估量的价值。

Jörg Wiltfang博士主任教授

口腔颌面外科

德国Schleswig-Holstein大学医学中心

Foreword (2)

This book has been written by Dr. Dr. Yu Jianmin. Dr. Yu has studied and worked at Chinese Medical University in Shenyang. This institution is especially famous for its anatomical institute and the excellent teaching staff which has developed the "Chinese Flap". As a student, Dr. Yu was able to profit from this experience and also contributed drawings to various works after finishing his degrees.

He is a brilliant reconstructive surgeon with profound knowledge in craniofacial anatomy. Besides these outstanding surgical skills, he is an artist and able to create excellent anatomic drawings. His profound knowledge of the anatomy of the human being, his excellent surgical experience and his artistic skills are united in this textbook of lower lip reconstruction.

Besides traumatology, lip cancer is one of the main reasons for lower lip deficiencies. Achieving a favourable aesthetic and functional outcome is the prerequisite for high life quality following this kind of surgery.

Dr. Yu gives a review of 192 years and 96 methods of lower lip reconstruction. Following the introduction, the anatomy of the perioral region is shown. After giving a survey of the possibilities of lip reconstruction with direct approximation, advancement flaps, rotation flaps and distant flaps, Dr. Yu shows his methods of lower lip reconstruction, giving very valuable hints for this kind of surgery. His surgical procedures are illustrated by excellent drawing and descriptions of the methods.

The book is written in Chinese and English in an intelligible and unambiguous language and thus can be read in a simple and quick way. For better comprehensibility, operated access paths and procedures are illustrated by excellent drawing in large numbers. In conclusion, this book is a very valuable edition for every colleague dealing with reconstructive surgery, especially with lower lip reconstruction.

All in all, this book is full of treasures for our colleagues.

Director Prof. Dr. Dr. Jörg Wiltfang

Department of Oral and Maxillofacial Surgery

University Medical Center Schleswig-Holstein

著者前言

本书中我运用大量插图总结阐述了我自己研创的下唇再造技术。这也是我在德国弗里德里希–亚历山大–埃朗根–纽伦堡大学医学院博士论文课题研究的主要内容。为尽可能保证整篇著作毫无错漏，我进行了详细的资料检索。希望从口腔颌面外科、整容及一般外科角度在下唇再造方面提供理想的帮助。

任何领域新技术的开发都需要基础知识构建的坚实基础。对于每一位医学研究者来说，人类解剖学这一学科就是其专业领域中最重要的组成部分。著名的"中国皮瓣"是由沈阳中国医科大学的解剖学李吉教授和陆军总院外科杨果凡医生研究和发明的。手术需要先通过特殊的方式灌注一种液体来使前臂的血管明显变红可见。然后通过复杂而费时的过程将血管从周围分离。当除去所有其他结缔组织之后就可以得到纯粹的前臂血管网。显微血管外科杨医生可以通过桡动脉或尺动脉和其伴随的静脉创建带蒂皮瓣并成功运用于显微血管外科。关于此技术的文章也在医学专业杂志上发表。这一前臂皮瓣也被正式命名为"中国皮瓣"。1976年在我写作《实用解剖图谱》的工作过程中，有幸与李教授有过接触。他向我展示了前臂血管网–血管铸型。我亲眼目睹了这一极富魅力的工艺品，并被其深深打动且留下深刻印象。今天，"中国皮瓣"是在医学领域唯一被冠以"中国"字样的专有名词，这是沈阳中国医科大学的骄傲。如果没有李教授在解剖学方面全面的知识，"中国皮瓣"就不可能研发成功。当时这也使我意识到必须努力学习人体解剖学才能成为一名优秀的外科医生。我当时用心、细心地投入，为以后研发下唇再造新技术打下了坚实的基础。

在此我要衷心感谢加拿大魁北克省蒙特利尔St.Mary's医院的Mercier教授。他在1987年和1988年希望我去加拿大和他一起进行一部或多部世界级专业图谱的编制。为此他4次向我发出书面邀请，并2次来德国与我就此工作进行面谈。向我详细介绍了魁北克的风土人情，并希望我能够和他一起在蒙特利尔共事5年。但当时由于我无法在加拿大从事外科医生的工作，只得很遗憾地拒绝了他的邀请。虽然时间过去很久，但直到今天我还是从心里对Mercier教授充满无尽感激。感谢他对于我艺术和专业方面能力的高度认可和对于我人品方面的充分肯定。希望如果他能看到我的这本著作，能理解我当时的处境和做出的决定。

余健民

Editor's Words

In this book, I have comprehensively presented my new technique of lower lip reconstruction with the help of figures. This work was the essential part of my dissertation submitted for the fulfillment of the requirements for the doctoral degree at the Faculty of Medicine of the Friedrich-Alexander-University of Erlangen-Nuremberg in Germany. For this, I have conducted an in-depth literature research to compose a complete work. I hope that this book presents an ideal aid for oral and maxillofacial surgeons, plastic and general surgeons when performing lower lip reconstructions.

In every field, the development of a new technique demands a solid foundation of basic knowledge. The study of human anatomy is the most important part of their profession for every physician. The famous "Chinese Flap" was researched and developed in Shenyang by Professor for Anatomy Mr. Li Ji of the Chinese Medical University and the surgeon Mr. Yang Guofan of the main clinic of the ground forces. Using a specific method, a liquid was injected to visualize the vessels of the forearm in a distinct red color. Then, the blood vessels were extracted from their environment by means of a complicated and laborious procedure. After removal of all other parts of the tissue, the pure blood vessel system could be displayed. From the arteria radialis and the accompanying vein, or the arteria ulnaris and the accompanying vein, the microvascular surgeon Yang could form a flap pedicle that was successfully used in microvascular surgery. An article on this technique was published in a medical journal. This forearm flap is officially called "Chinese Flap". While I was working on the *Atlas for Practical Anatomy* in 1976, I was fortunate to be in touch with Professor Li. Professor Li showed me the specimen of the vessel network casting mold of the forearm. To see this magnificent work of art with my own eyes, I was deeply moving and had a deep impression. Today, the "Chinese Flap" is the only term in the medical field that puts "China" first. It is the pride and joy of the Chinese Medical University in Shenyang. The "Chinese Flap" could only become so famous because Professor Li had comprehensive knowledge of anatomy. Even back then I knew that I had to study the human anatomy accurately to become a good surgeon. With meticulous commitment I was able to lay the foundation for developing a new lower lip reconstruction technique.

At this point, I want to give my sincere thanks to Professor Mercier of St. Mary's hospital in Montréal, Quebec. In 1987 and 1988, it was Professor Mercier's wish that together in Canada, he and I would create one or more professional atlases on world-class level. He sent me 4 invitation letters and travelled to Germany twice to talk to me personally. He explained to me in detail the local conditions and the mentality in Quebec. He was hoping to win me over for a five-year cooperation in Montréal. Much to my regret, I had to decline this offer as I couldn't have worked as a surgeon there. But in my heart, I am still very grateful that Professor Mercier highly valued my artistic and professional abilities and had put great trust in me. Even though many years have passed, I am eternally grateful to this day. I hope that Professor Mercier will understand my motives and decisions after reading this book.

Yu Jianmin

简介

唇癌是介于口腔癌和皮肤癌之间的一种癌症。它多发于口周围皮肤和口腔黏膜的移行区域，即所谓边缘区。

唇癌多发于60~70岁的男性人群，而其中90%发生于下唇。患者以农村人口和社会中下层人士为主。引发病变的主要诱因是外源性的氮氧化物。首先要讨论的是气候因素，特别是太阳辐射。另一个引发癌变的因素是温度和化学的刺激，其主要来源于吸烟形成的蒸馏产物。唇癌尤其多发于唇部边缘中间或嘴角。其早期症状表现为组织肿大、过度角化以及相对应的表面呈乳头状覆盖的唇黏膜肿胀。还有可能表现为发展成溃疡的黏膜表面的侵蚀性变化（表面溃烂）。病程进展在宏观上可分为外生型和内生型两种。外生型多表现为乳头状增生，而内生型则主要表现为深层细胞组织的肿大和硬化以及部分溃烂。这两种病程进展多数情况下相互伴生，进而形成相类似的深度溃疡，周边硬化，边缘外翻高低不平的不均匀突起。由于溃疡的易感染性，使得对于淋巴结区域的临床评估比较困难。基本上表现为溃烂和浸润的病程进展型癌症比外生型病程进展的癌症更易于转移。相对于其他口腔癌症，唇癌发展较慢。根据统计，从发病到扩散至淋巴结平均病程为2年。转移的发生率低，一般会随着原发肿瘤的大小和病理组织后期分化程度而增加。基于所有T类别转移发生率在6%~14%，对于邻近淋巴结转移的治疗诊断存在不同的看法。一些作者由于原发性唇癌相对较低的淋巴结转移发生率，把临床怀疑现有的潜在的颈部淋巴结转移作为实施颈淋巴结根治性切除术的适应证，其他人则建议起码对于T2和T3型肿瘤基本上应实施预防性选择性颈部舌骨上区清除术。

98%发生于唇部的鳞状细胞癌是在下唇，这表明下唇癌的产生与环境因素中的光照直接相关。基底细胞癌与其相反，多发生于上唇。值得注意的是，发生于上唇的鳞状细胞癌虽然极少出现，却往往会在早期出现转移。很少在下唇部位发现唾液腺癌、黑色素瘤和肉瘤。和其他口腔癌症比较，下唇癌的诊断尤为便利准确。不考虑T分类系统，唇癌的5年治愈率公认为70%。绝大多数笔者对于原发性肿瘤的治疗相比放射性治疗更偏好于外科手术治疗。可采取的手术介入有：

1. 初期采取简单的楔形切除，创口直接愈合；

2. 当肿瘤大于1cm，切除并采取预防性措施，或选择同侧或双侧舌骨上淋巴结清除术；

3. 肿瘤转移至颈上淋巴结，切除同时实施同侧颈部淋巴结清除术。

在埃朗根口腔颌面外科医院，根据经验一般施行舌骨上淋巴结清扫术，当被证明出现淋巴结转移的情况时则扩大为单侧或双侧颈部淋巴结清除术。如果下唇的缺损超过下唇部的30%，大面积的缺损通过再造整容手术是必要的。

下唇再造的手术技术异常丰富，有些已有200多年历史。这些手术分为：直接缝合、邻近皮瓣和远位皮瓣。邻近皮瓣可分为：推进皮瓣、旋转皮瓣或两者相结合的皮瓣。

Abstract

Cancer of the lip holds a position between cancer of the oral cavity and skin cancer. Lip carcinomas generally begin in the region where the white area of the lip borders on the oral mucosa; this is the so-called vermilion border of the lip.

Men above 60 or 70 years of age are especially prone to carcinoma of the lip and in over 90% of cases it is the lower lip which is affected. The majority of patients are from rural populations and from the lower and middle social classes. In etiological terms, exogenous noxae play a deciding role. Climatic influences, especially exposure to the sun are in the focus of discussion. Further oncogenic factors are thermal and chemical irritation caused by the distillates resulting from smoking. Lip carcinoma occurrence is principally paramedian in the lipborder area or in the corner of the mouth. Early symptoms are a thickening of tissue, hyperkeratosis or papillary, scabby distension of the labial mucosa. Also possible are erosive changes in the mucosal surface which deteriorate to an ulcer. Macroscopically, exophytic and endophytic growth types can be distinguished. Growth of the exophytic type generally manifests as a papillomatous tumor while the endophytic type manifests as a primary thickening and induration of the deeper tissue layers, which then secondarily ulcerates. Often, both pathogeneses occur together. In the late stage the appearance is nearly identical: a deep ulcer with an indurated environment and distended, irregular margins. Because ulcers of this type may become superinfected, it is difficult to clinically assess the lymph node area. In principle, primary ulcerous carcinomas with an infiltrating growth pattern are more prone to metastasis than carcinomas which grow exophytically. The growth rate of lip carcinomas tends to be slower than that of other carcinomas of the oral cavity. Statistical studies have shown that lymphnode metastasis occurs on an average of two years after the beginning of the disease. The metastasis frequency is low but according to general findings increases with growth of the primary tumour and the pathohistologic degree of differentiation (STEIGLEDER, 1974) and is about 6% and 14% based on all T categories. Opinions about prognostic consequences of a therapy of the bordering lymphatic drainage system differ. Because of a relatively low incidence of lymphnode metastasis after primary lip carcinoma, some authors consider that a radical neck dissection is indicated only if there is clinical suspicion of preexisting neck lymphnode metastasis. Others recommend preventive or elective emptying of the suprahyoid region of the neck as mainstay, providing the tumors are T2 or T3.

In 98% of all cases, squamouscell carcinomas of the lip occur in the lower lip. There appears to be a direct link between exposure to environmental influences and the causation of lower lip cancer. In contrast, basalcell cancers are found mainly in the upper lip. It is noteworthy that the less commonly occurring squamouscell carcinomas of the upper lip show a disposition to earlier metastasis. Cancer of the salivary gland as well as melanomas and sarcomas have rarely been observed in the labial region. Prognosis of lower lip carcinomas is assessed as being considerably more favorable than that of other types of cancer of the oral cavity. A 5-year survival rate of 70% is assumed for lip cancer regardless of its T classification. In the literature, the vast majority of authors agree that surgical treatment of the primary tumor is preferable to radiological treatment. The following operative options exist:

1. simple wedge excision and primary adaptation of the wound edges in the early stages;

2. excision and preventive or elective homolateral or bilateral suprahyoid lymph node dissection when the tumor measures over 1 cm;

3. excision and ipsilateral neck dissection in the upper neck lymph nodes if metastasis has occurred.

In our experience at the Maxillofacial Clinic of Erlangen, suprahyoid lymph node dissection is carried out as a rule for diagnostic purposes. If lymph node metastasis is hereby discovered, surgery is then extended to neck dissection on one or both sides. If the defect of the lower lip involves over 30% of the labial area, primary defect coverage by means of reconstructive plastic surgery is indicated.

A remarkably high number of operative techniques for lower lip reconstruction exist, some of which are as old as 200 years. These operations are classified: direct approximation, those using local flaps for reconstruction and those using distant flaps. Within the local flap category, the following techniques can be distinguished: advancement flaps, rotation flaps and combinations of both.

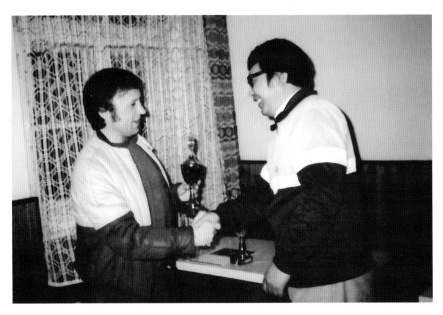

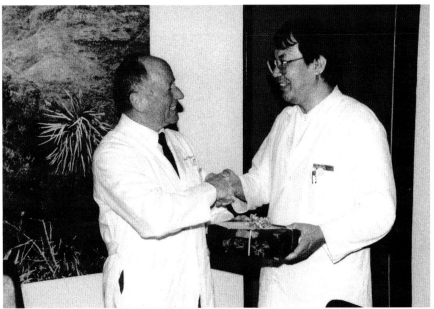

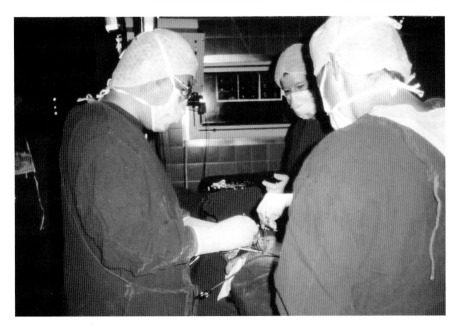

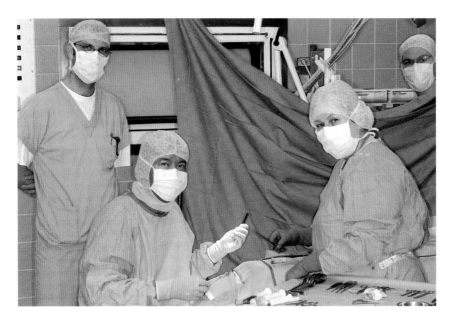

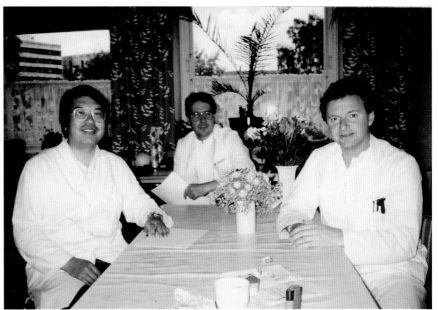

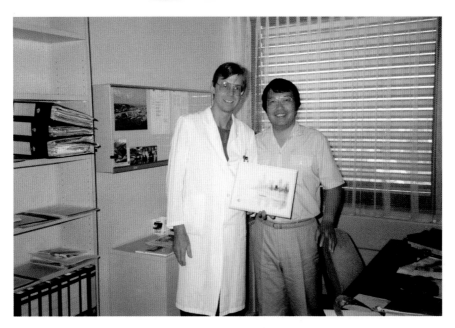

目录 Contents

第**1**章

Chapter 1

口周围解剖

The Anatomy of the Perioral Region

口腔周边软组织由皮肤、黏膜、皮下组织、肌肉、神经血管和唾液腺组成。作为身体筋膜的浅筋膜，分隔于皮下区域和其下部的肌肉之间，从舌骨延伸到下颌骨，从胸锁乳突肌前缘延伸到下颌角及颧弓。在下颌角的高度，浅筋膜分为两层，作为咬肌筋膜包裹住咬肌和翼内肌。咬肌筋膜终止于外侧咀嚼肌内侧边缘，因此在张口区域的面部表情肌是没有筋膜的。

The soft tissue in the vicinity of the oral fissure consists of skin, mucosa, subcutaneous tissue, muscles, nerve vessels and salivary glands. The fascia superficialis, a body tissue which separates the subcutaneous region from the underlying muscle, extends from the hyoid to the mandible and from the anterior edge of the sternocleidomastoid to the mandibular angle and the zygomatic arch. Level with the mandibular angle, the fascia superficialis divides into two sheets: as the masseteric fascia it encases the masseter muscle and the medial pterygoid muscle. The masseteric fascia inserts at the medial edge of the outer masseter muscle, so the mimetic muscles in the region of the oral opening have no fasciae.

眼角和嘴角的皱纹是细胞组织老化的标志。在此区域存在着匝肌，它通过持续地收缩周边毗邻的组织来支撑起皮肤，从而改变皮肤与其下肌肉的附着。当此肌肉群过度疲劳并伴随着皮下组织的萎缩，就会首先引起相应部位皮肤表层的变化。肌肉、表层筋膜、皮下组织及脂肪在脸部互相连接，组成一个功能单元。为了理解口周和眼周皮肤皱纹的形成，必须了解表情肌的功能。表情肌组成了由面第七对脑神经控制的单元。其中口轮匝肌主要负责口、唇及毗邻脸颊肌肉群的运动。相毗邻的肌肉和相邻的肌肉群被相邻的脂肪组织和浅筋膜包裹交织。特别是在口周围区域筋膜和肌肉通过互相交织形成了一个完整的单元。这就使得此肌肉群既有由于情感刺激而表达表情的作用，同时也有生理功能，从而导致其不可避免在皮肤表面形成皱纹。

Signs of tissue-aging are manifested mainly in the formation of furrows and wrinkles at the eyes and corners of the mouth. As a result of continual contraction of the adjacent tissue, the orbicular muscle present in this area raises the skin, thus changing the adherence between the skin and its underlying muscle. Together with atrophy of the subcutaneous tissue in this region, overwear of these muscle groups leads to initial changes in the skin's surface. In the facial area, muscles, superficial tissue, subcutaneous tissue and fat are interconnected in such a manner that they form a functional unit. In order to understand perioral and periorbital formation of skin wrinkles, we must take the function of the mimetic muscles into consideration. These muscles form a unit which is controlled by the facial nerve (VII. Cranial Nerve). When performing reconstructive measures in the face, this contractile network of muscles must be taken into consideration. The orbicularis oris muscle is primarily responsible for movement of the mouth, the lips and the adjacent cheek muscles. The adjacent muscles interweave the neighboring adipose tissue and the subcutaneous fasciae, and, in many places, also the neigh-boring muscles. Interspersion of fasciae and muscle to the extent of forming a complete unit is especially manifest in the perioral region. This is why these muscle groups express emotions and complete physiological tasks. As a consequence, their contraction inevitably causes a pattern of wrinkles and furrows.

1. 口周围肌肉群

口周区域肌肉分为环状收缩肌，口轮匝肌和位于口唇周边的可上提上唇、降下唇或拉口角向上、向下或向外的辐射状肌肉。口轮匝肌组成了唇的基本肌肉结构。它是由横向圆弧形不同方向的肌纤维在上下唇区域组成，集中经过嘴角，其中部分通过神经延伸入皮肤并过渡进入周边肌肉群。在唇红区域，口轮匝肌肌肉边缘向前扩散，被称为口轮匝肌唇部。作为占环状肌多数的口轮匝肌缘部，在皮下区域扩展至梨状沟及靠近颏隆凸。下颌部的环肌则被下唇降肌穿过并部分被其覆盖。整个肌肉通过其向外侧倾斜拉伸的纤维与真皮相附着。通过这种连接，使皮肤能够跟随环肌的各种动作变化，很大程度上使唇能够做出各种口形。

1. Perioral Muscles

In the perioral region, we distinguish the circular sphincter muscle, the so-called orbicularis oris and the dilator muscles of the oral fissure, which extend radially into the neighboring region. The orbicularis oris muscle forms the fundamental muscular structure of the lip. This muscle is made up of obliquely running, arched muscle fiber in the region of the upper and lower lips. The muscle fibers decussate laterally at the corners of the mouth. By means of tendons, the orbicularis oris muscle partially inserts into the epidermis and merges with the surrounding muscle. In the region of the lip vermilion the contours of the orbicularis oris muscle curl outward to form a marginal protrusion; this part is the so-called pars labialis. The main part of the circular muscle, the pars marginalis, is flat and spreads beneath the epidermis up to the piriform aperture and up to the vicinity of the mental protuberance. The depressor labii inferioris muscle inserts into and partially covers the mandibular part of the circular muscle. The entire orbicularis oris muscle is attached to the corium by oblique, outwardly running fibers. This permits the skin to follow the variable play of the ring muscle, thus allowing varying forms of the lip.

口轮匝肌与皮肤的连接要强于与黏膜的连接。皮肤结缔组织延伸入肌肉纤维间，从而使皮肤与其下的口轮匝肌形成牢固的连接。皮肤与肌肉间的这种固定连接赋予了唇的许多个性特点动作及共性。唇实现各种动作，如说话、吮吸、吹口哨及吹奏所需要的形状变化，很难用力学理论来理解，结缔组织与肌肉组织间的交错连接可以使这种变形成为可能。口轮匝肌的主要功能是关闭口裂。通过唇边缘的进一步细微调整可使唇缘做出嘟嘴、噘起的动作。噘嘴的形成主要通过口轮匝肌唇部放松时的边缘部来实现。另外，肌纤维止于鼻尖软骨，使鼻中隔通过鼻中隔降肌向下运动。

The orbicularis oris muscle is more firmly connected with the skin than with the mucosa. The subcutaneous connective tissue of the skin inserts between the muscle fibers and it forms a strong connection between the overlying skin and the underlying orbicularis oris muscle. This firm connection between skin and muscle lends the lips their specific, individual, pursed form. The interspersion of connective tissue with muscle enables mechanically complex changes in lip form such as are required for speaking, sucking, whistling, blowing, etc. The prominent function of the orbicularis oris muscle consists in closing the orifice of the mouth. Furthermore, the labial parts of the orbicularis oris muscle enable the fine lip movements involved in inwardly rolling and pursing the lips. Rolling the lip margin outwardly is enabled principally by the marginal parts of the orbicularis oris muscle, whereby the labial part is relaxed. Further muscle fibers insert in the cartilage of the nasal tip and can move the nasal septum in a caudal direction by means of the depressor septi nasi muscle.

2. 上唇鼻翼提肌

上颌骨内侧的上唇鼻翼提肌是上唇鼻内侧提肌，从鼻梁靠近内侧眼角处向下外并延伸至鼻区和人中部皮肤。它的功能是开大鼻孔和人中向上，由此来提升上唇，同时它也与从内侧眼角向鼻梁方向的皱纹有关。

2. Levator labii superioris alaeque nasi muscle

The levator nasi et labii maxillaris medialis, the medial elevator muscle of the nose and upper lip arises from the bridge of the nose in the vicinity of the medial canthus and inserts on the region of the ala of the nose and the dermis of the philtrum. Its function consists in dilating the nostril and elevating the philtrum, causing the lip to lift. At the same time, it is responsible for the formation of wrinkles running from the medial canthus to the bridge of the nose.

上唇提肌是鼻子和上唇的外侧提升装置，从眶下孔上部向下，下行至鼻翼和鼻唇沟，其作用是通过向上牵拉鼻子来提升上唇和开大鼻孔。

The superior levator labii muscle, which is the lateral elevator muscle of the nose and upper lip, arises superior to the infraorbital foramen and inserts on the wing of the nose and the nasolabial groove and elevates the nose, together with the upper lip and is also responsible for the dilation of the nostril.

颧小肌是一块小颧骨肌肉。它起于颧骨下行至鼻唇沟皮肤，从颧大肌内侧嵌入上唇。它的作用是向外和向颅侧牵拉嘴角。

The zygomaticus minor muscle, the small cheek-bone muscle, arises from the zygoma and inserts on the skin of the nasolabial groove. The muscle inserts medially on the zygomaticus major in the upper lip. Its function consists in lateral and cranial elevation of the commissure of the mouth.

颧大肌是一块大颧骨肌肉。它起自颧骨外表面和颧骨颧颞缝，斜向下外延伸至口轮匝肌中缝以及周边皮肤和黏膜。颧大肌属于笑肌，通过颧大肌的收缩可以把嘴角向侧上方牵引，同时鼻唇沟同样向侧上方移动，从而使鼻唇沟的皮肤隆起。

The zygomaticus major, or greater zygomatic muscle, arises from the lateral surface of the zygomatic bone and from the zygomaticotemporal suture line. It inserts obliquely on the raphe of the orbicularis oris and on the adjacent dermis and mucosa. When contracted, this muscle elevates and laterally moves the commissure. This makes it the actual laughing muscle. At the same time, the nasolabial groove is pushed cranially in a lateral direction, thus enabling the skin in the region of the nasolabial fold to protrude when this muscle is in action.

口角提肌即尖牙肌，起自眶下孔下部尖牙窝，延伸至口轮匝肌及三角肌。它的功能是上提嘴角。

The caninus, or levator anguli oris muscle arises beneath the infraorbital foramen, in the canine fossa and inserts to the orbicularis oris and triangular muscles. It also functions to superiorly elevate the commissure.

笑肌，事实上是口角降肌边缘一部分。它从侧面牵拉嘴角，即从口轮匝肌缝向后分散到脸颊皮肤。这个走行的变量非常大，它既能倾向于尾部，也能倾向于颅侧或只形成于单侧。

The risorius muscle is in reality a lateral branch of the depressor anguli oris muscle. It retracts from the lateral commissure, that is, from the raphe of the orbicularis oris muscle to the dermis of the cheek. Its course can be exceptionally diverse. It can run caudally as well as in a slightly cranial direction. In addition, it can be developed only unilaterally.

当笑肌收缩时，可使脸颊皮肤向嘴角方向移动，从而在微笑时脸颊皮肤能够向内打褶并收缩形成所谓的酒窝。当肌肉纤维向外侧向腮腺筋膜移动，可使嘴角向背向移动。此时它的功能与颊肌类似。这种情况下，肌肉的收缩不会产生酒窝。

Upon contraction of this muscle, the buccal dermis is shifted towards the commissure, so that laughter folds the buccal dermis inwardly and retracts it, producing dimples. If the muscle fibers course laterally, in the direction of the parotid fascia, the commissure is shifted dorsally, somewhat like in the functioning of the buccinator muscle. In this case, contraction of the muscle does not produce dimples.

口角降肌即三角肌。它起于下颌下缘，颅向汇集于嘴角并在嘴角处嵌入皮肤。当口角降肌收缩时，可使嘴角向下移动，并展平鼻唇沟上弧线。

The depressor anguli oris muscle, or the triangular muscle, arises from the inferior margin of the mandible, converges cranially to the commissure and inserts there on the dermis. Upon contraction, a caudal shift of the commissure and flattening of the superior arch of the nasolabial groove occur.

下唇降肌即下唇方肌。它起于下颌基部，扇形延伸入口轮匝肌。下唇降肌的功能是向下牵拉下唇。

The depressor labii inferioris or quadrate muscle of the lower lip arises from the base of the mandible and inserts in a fan shape to the orbicularis oris muscle. In action it depresses the lower lip.

颊肌为颊部肌肉，它起于上下颌骨磨牙牙槽突的外面和翼突下颌缝。翼突下颌缝为下颌骨与翼钩之间的致密结缔组织，同时也是咽上缩肌的起源部分。颊肌下部分纤维颅侧弧形拉伸并延伸至上唇口轮匝肌，上部分纤维弧形拉伸向下延伸至下唇。纤维于口角外侧交叉并在此形成可觉察甚至有时可见的膨胀部分。颊肌是膨胀的主要部分，与口轮匝肌共同作用下，可缩小牙列与脸颊及嘴唇间距离，即缩小口腔前庭。由此饮食是通过咀嚼动作将食物从口腔前庭位置送回咀嚼区域。颊部脂肪垫位于颊肌后部与咬肌之间，这一脂肪组织提供了可变形的滑动层并给予脸颊以巨大的支撑，它对于吮吸动作具有重要意义。当恶病质时颊脂垫会出现萎缩。

The buccinator or cheek muscle arises from the alveolar process of the upper and lower jaw-bones in the region of the last molars and the pterygomandibular raphe, a strip of connective tissue, stretched out between the lower jaw and the pterygoid hamulus. The pterygomandibular raphe also serves as the origin of parts of the superior pharyngeal constrictor. The inferior fibers of the buccinator muscle rise cranially in an arch and insert on the orbicularis muscle of the upper lip; the superior fibers descend in an arch and insert to the lower lip. Its fibers intersect lateral to the commissure, where they form the main part of a clearly palpable and occasionally even visible distension. This muscle forms the fundament of the curvature of the cheek. In conjunction with the orbicularis oris muscle, it reduces the opening of the oral vestibule, the area between the teeth, and cheeks or lips, thus moving food during eating and chewing from the region of the oral vestibule back to the masticatory surface. The buccal fat-pad, or corpus adiposum buccae is situated between the posterior part of the buccinator muscle and the masseter muscle. This fat-pad provides a malleable, gliding surface and lends certain stability to the cheek. It is said to play a significant role in enabling sucking. Atrophy of this fat pad occurs only in cachexia.

颏肌即下颌肌肉，它起于下颌骨侧切牙的牙槽突的骨面，放散式行向下内，部分与口角降肌相交叉止于颏结节，直到越过中线对侧之区域的颏部皮肤。

The mentalis, or chin muscle, arises from the alveolar jugulum of the inferior lateral incisors, diverges medially in a downward direction, partially traverses the depressor anguli oris muscle and inserts to the dermis of the chin from the region of the mental tubercle, crossing over the median to the opposite side.

3. 口周的血管供应

口周区域主要由面动脉的分支血管来供应。作为颈外动脉的第三分支的面动脉，起自主血管的舌动脉上方。经过二腹肌内侧与茎突舌骨肌迂回曲折至颌下腺窝，经过下颌下腺上方沟内，在下颌下方与颏下动脉紧密缠绕。颏下动脉在二腹肌和下颌舌骨肌之间前行。面动脉继续在嘴角处曲折经过颊肌，抵达眼角内侧成为内眦动脉，内眦动脉在内眦部与颈内动脉的分支眼动脉的一支鼻外动脉有吻合。面动脉在向内眦运程中释放出许多分支，包括上下唇动脉。此外还与颏动脉、眶下动脉、颊动脉和面横动脉有吻合。面静脉伴行于动脉并基本上具有同名血管，它作为内眦静脉起自眼角内侧的滑车上静脉和眶上静脉。这两条静脉直接与眼静脉上支相连。面静脉在面部的进程中，于鼻外侧会合鼻外静脉、上唇处的上唇静脉、脸颊后部和翼丛的面深静脉、颊部的腮静脉，以及下唇的下唇静脉。面静脉继续环绕下颌基部，与动脉并行且在口底下侧与颏下静脉会合。

3. Blood supply to the oral region

The blood supply to the perioral region stems primarily from branches of the facial artery. The facial artery, the third branch of the external carotid system, ramifies from its main artery above the lingual artery. It passes in an arch above the medial side of the digastric and stylohyoideus muscle into the submandibular fossa, runs along a groove superior to the submandibular gland, and drains right beneath the mandible into the submental artery, which has an anterior path between the digastric and mylohyoid muscle. The facial artery continues in a winding course above the buccinator muscle, passes the commissure, and ends at the medial canthus as the arteria angularis. Here, it anastomoses with the dorsal nasal artery, a branch of the ophthalmic artery from the internal carotid artery. Along its way to the canthus it divides into numerous branches, the most important of which are the inferior and superior labial arteries. Further anastomoses take place with the mental, infraorbital and buccal arteries, as well as the transversa faciei. The facial vein accompanies the facial artery and contains branches with essentially the same names. The facial vein originates at the medial canthus as the angular vein from the supratrochlear and supraorbital veins. Both of the latter veins are directly connected with the superior ophthalmic vein. During its course on the face, the facial vein receives the external nasal veins of the ala nasi, the superior labial vein of the upper lip, the deep facial vein of the depths of the cheek and the pterygoid venous plexus, the parotid veins of the parotid, as well as the inferior labial vein of the lower lip. The facial vein then circumvents the base of the lower maxilla dorsally to the artery, and receives the submental vein at the underside of the floor of the mouth.

4. 淋巴分布关系

面部的淋巴管主要与血管相关。淋巴管主要注入颏下淋巴结和下颌下淋巴结。癌症病灶越靠近腹侧，则第一个过滤站首先被侵袭的概率就越大。对于唇癌，颏下和下颌下区域淋巴结几乎90%被累及。然而，会有变异的颈前淋巴结链将颏下淋巴结与内侧和尾侧的颈淋巴结短路连接。这种与主流方向相差异的转移途径在所有情况中占到11%。综上所述得出，舌骨淋巴结清扫术将会发现触诊发觉不到的大多数细小的淋巴转移。

4. Lymphatic Drainage

The regional lymph vessels of the facial region run mainly in relationship to the blood vessels. The draining lymph vessels coalesce primarily in the submental and submandibular lymph nodes. The more ventral the location of a carcinoma, the greater the probability, that the first filter will be affected first. First echelon nodes for carcinomas of the lip are the mental and submandibular lymph nodes in almost 90%. However, it may occur that an inconstant anterior cervical chain of lymph nodes bypasses the submental lymph nodes with the medial and caudal jugular lymph nodes. This path of metastasis deviates from the main and occurs in some 11%. This information makes it clear, that performance of a suprahyoid lymph node dissection will detect by far the largest part of micrometastases which are not discernible through palpation.

5. 口周神经分布

口周区域的主要神经是三叉神经的感觉支。上唇由眶下神经（V2）末支支配，下唇区域由颏神经（V3）末支支配。与面神经末支相比，面部三叉神经分布更深更隐蔽。眶下神经从眶下孔穿出，位于颧上颌裂约0.8cm处表面。从那里开始分布于尖牙窝、鼻和上唇。颏神经（V3）由下颌管第二前磨牙高度处向下唇和颏区域分布。

5. Innervation of the perioral region

The principal nerves in the periorbital region are sensitive branches of the trigeminal nerve. The upper lip is innervated by terminal branches of the infraorbital nerve (V2), the lower lip region by terminal branches of the mental nerve (V3). Contrary to the terminal branches of the facial nerve, the sensitive trigeminal branches of the facial region lie deeper and are hidden. The infraorbital nerve surfaces at the infraorbital foramen, approximately 0.8 cm beneath the zygomaticomaxillary fissure. From there, the nerves diverge in the canine fossa in a fan shape to reach the nose and upper lip. Branches of the mental nerve (V3) ramify from the mandibular canal, level with the second premolars, and diverge in a fan shape in the lower lip and chin area.

脸部表情肌由面神经支配，面神经从茎乳孔穿出并分布于脸部。它在唾液腺内形成位于多层纤维隔中的腮腺丛，腮腺被面神经分为表层和深层两部分。在腮腺前缘，面神经明确分支至表面，横向放射状穿过面部中间区域，下行进入面部表情肌。

The mimetic facial muscles are innervated by the facial nerve. The facial nerve exits the stylomastoid foramen and diverges into the facial region. Inside the parotid gland, the facial nerve forms the parotid plexus, which lies within an areal septum of connective tissue. The parotid gland is partly divided into a superficial and a deep part by the facial nerve. The branches of the facial nerve surface manifestly at the anterior border of the parotid gland, then cross the medial part of the facial region radially and ascend to insert on the mimetic face muscles.

在所有唇部的再造手术操作中都要注意到这一解剖形态（图1.1～图1.5）。

The anatomic facts described above must be taken into consideration for all reconstructive operations in the area of the lips (Fig1.1~Fig1.5).

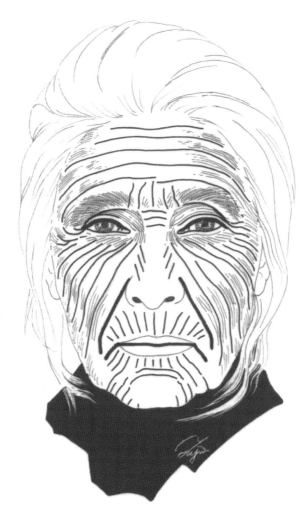

图1.1　面部皮肤纹

Fig. 1.1　Facial skin creases

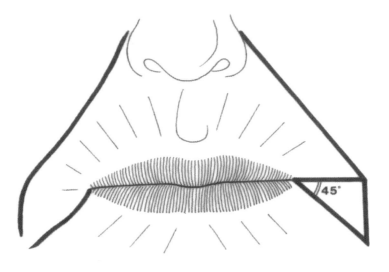

图1.2　鼻唇沟与嘴角区域纹

Fig. 1.2　The nasolabial groove and labiomandibular crease

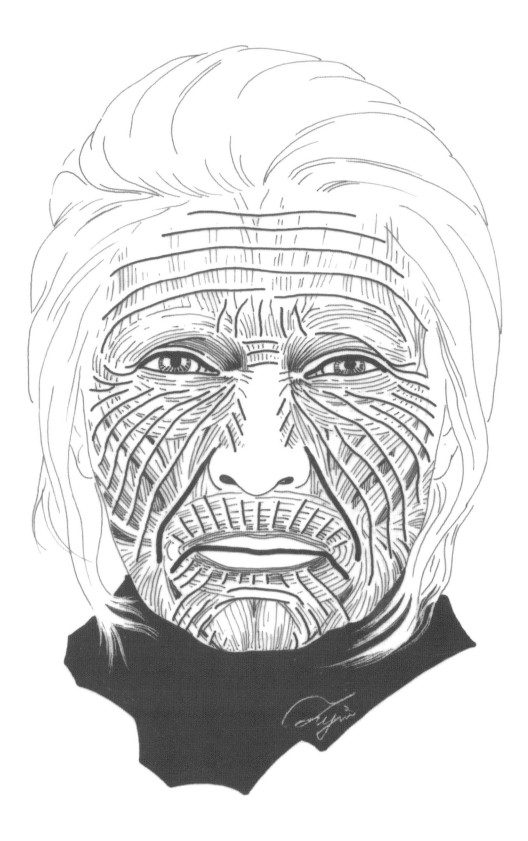

图1.3　皮肤纹与肌肉走向的关系

Fig. 1.3　Facial skin wrinkles in relation to the course of the muscles

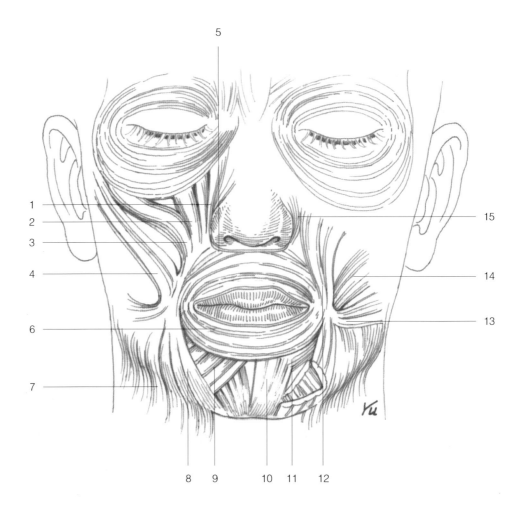

图1.4　口周围表情肌

Fig. 1.4　Mimetic muscles in the region of the mouth

1. 上唇鼻翼提肌　M. levator labii sup aleque nasi
2. 上唇提肌　M. levator labii sup
3. 颧小肌　M. zygomaticus minor
4. 颧大肌　M. zygomaticus major
5. 口轮匝肌（边缘部）　M. orbicularis oris (pars marginalis)
6. 口轮匝肌（唇部）　M. orbicularis (pars labialis)
7. 颈阔肌　platysma

8. 口角降肌（三角肌）　M. depressor anguli oris
9. 下唇降肌（下唇方肌）　M. depressor labii inf.
10. 颏肌　M. mentalis
11. 颏横肌　M. transv. menti
12. 口角提肌（尖牙肌）　M. levator anguli oris
13. 笑肌　M. risorius
14. 颊肌　M. buccinator
15. 鼻肌（横部）　M. nasalis (pars transv.)

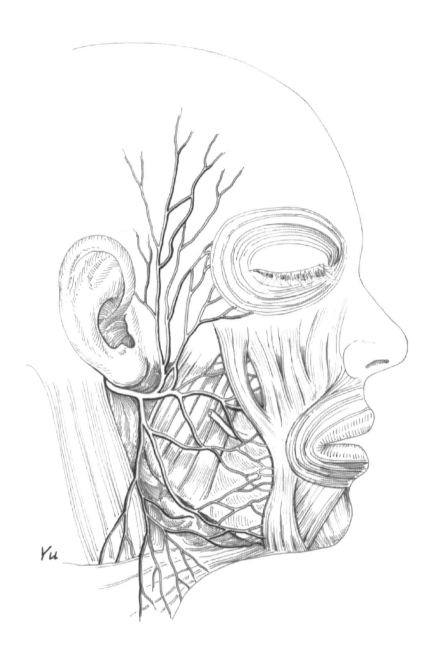

图1.5　面神经及其分支

Fig. 1.5　Facial nerve and its branches

第 **2** 章

Chapter 2

下唇再造术概论

A Survey of Lower Lip Reconstruction Procedures

以下将介绍95种下唇再造的方法。

In the following, 95 methods of lower lip reconstruction are described. These are classified from a plastic point of view:

根据整形的观点，分为直接缝合、推进皮瓣、旋转皮瓣、远位皮瓣。

Direct approximation– Advancement Flap - Rotational flap – Distant flap

1. 直接缝合

图2.1描绘切除下唇红病变的切口。图2.2描绘底层唇红的黏膜与其下方肌肉的分离。点线表示切除唇红部分的切口线。黏膜缺损通过缝合唇白边缘的前庭黏膜来修复。图2.3描绘了再造后缝合的效果。直径小于1cm的小肿瘤适用于楔形切除和创口直接愈合。图2.4描绘了V形切除下唇肿瘤。图2.5描绘了W形切除下唇肿瘤。创口的简单愈合保证了再造的可持续性。图2.6显示了W形切除下唇肿瘤后的最终形态。

1. Direct Approximation

Fig. 2.1 shows the incision for resection of a pathologically changed vermilion of the lower lip. Fig. 2.2 shows the mucous membrane being dissected off of the underlying muscle. The dotted line shows the line of incision for resection of a part of the lip vermilion. The mucosal defect can be closed by approximating the remaining vestibular mucous membrane to the margin of the white lip. Fig. 2.3 shows the result after reconstruction. For small tumors measuring less than 1 cm in diameter a wedge excision and primary adaptation of the wound margins are sufficient. Fig. 2.4 shows V-shaped resection of a tumor in the lower lip. Fig. 2.5 shows W-shaped resection of a malignant tumor in the lower lip. Restoration of continuity is achieved through simple adaptation of the wound edges. Fig. 2.6 depicts the final state after W-shaped resection of a lower lip tumor.

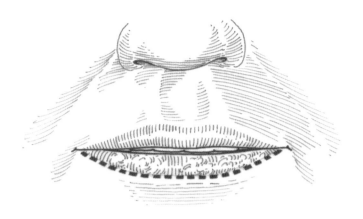

图2.1

Fig. 2.1

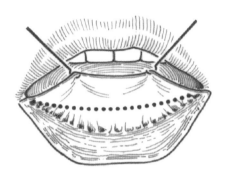

图2.2

Fig. 2.2

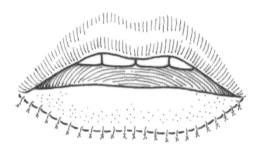

图2.3

Fig. 2.3

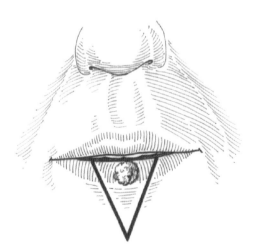

图2.4

Fig. 2.4

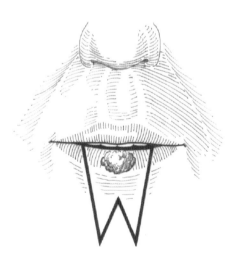

图2.5

Fig. 2.5

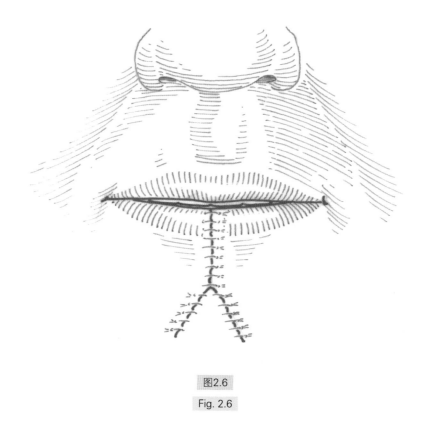

图2.6

Fig. 2.6

2. 推进皮瓣

在老的参考文献中，其中包括部分记载于19世纪的，记录了各种不同的通过改良推进皮瓣来实现的下唇再造修复方法。

2. Advancement Flaps

The older literature, some of which dates back as far as the nineteenth century, cites various methods of lip reconstruction using modified advancement flaps.

根据HORN方法（1860）或ROONHUYSEN方法（1870），肿瘤通过下唇的V形切口切除（图2.7-1）。根据肿瘤的大小，V形切口的顶端可向下延伸到颏下。此时V形切口的两边可能微微向外凹陷。从切口顶点沿下颌靠近下颌下缘创建1条或2条一指宽的切口，这样的松弛切口的创口可直接缝合。根据ROONHUYSEN的改进，为了扩展口裂，会在脸颊部额外创建两条贯穿所有三层组织的切口。先向上方外侧A-B，再向侧下方横向B-C。切口的终点（C点）位于嘴角（A）的高度位置。切口段A-B和B-C最后相缝合（图2.7-2）。由此下唇沿C-D-E扩展。唇内侧黏膜相应地切开更高，由此来创建唇红。这种方法不仅适用于唇中部的病变，同时也适用于侧面的病变。图2.7-3描绘了术后的最终形态。

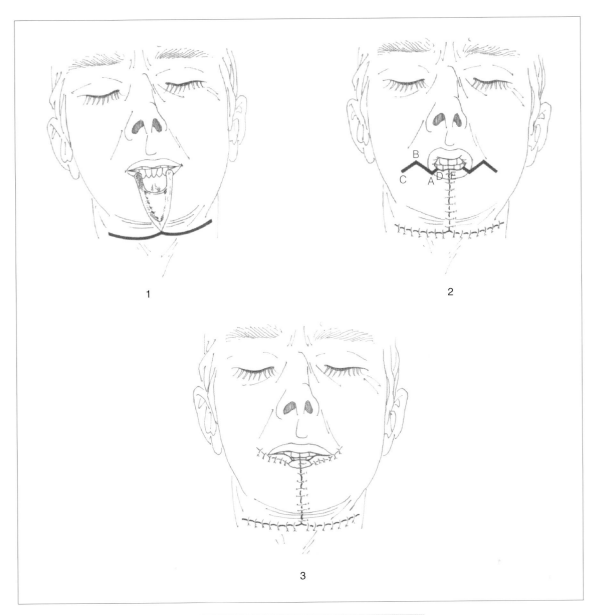

图2.7 HORN（1）和ROONHUYSEN（2.3）方法

Fig. 2.7 Method according to HORN(1) and ROONHUYSEN(2.3)

In the method according to HORN (1860) or ROONUYSEN (1870) the tumor is removed by means of a V-shaped incision in the region of the lower lip (Fig. 2.7-1). Depending on the size of the tumor, the point of the V-shaped excision can be extended as far as submentally. In this case, the sides of the V-shaped excision can be made slightly concave. One or two incisions are then made beginning from the point of the excision and running strictly submandibularly along the lower jaw-line one finger's width submandibular. This relaxing incision allows for a direct approximation of the wound edges. In a modified version according to ROONHUYSEN, two further incisions are made through all three thicknesses of the cheek, first upwards and outwards (A-B) and then downwards and laterally (B-C) in order to widen the orifice of the mouth. The end of the incision (point C) should be level with the commis-sure of the mouth (A). The line A-B is then sutured with the line B-C (Fig. 2.7-2). In this manner, the lower lip is widened by the length of C-D-E. Correspondingly, the mucosa of the inner side of the lip is circumcised on a slightly higher level, so that new lip vermilion can be formed. This method can be used for medially as well as laterally located lip defects. Fig. 2.7-3 shows the final result.

CELSE方法

这种方法是用矩形切口切除下唇病变的部分。通过一个水平的松弛切口在颊龈形成两个可以直接缝合的推进皮瓣。作为辅助，可以在面颊区域作两个额外的垂直的弧形辅助切口，其可在下唇残端缝合后延期封闭（图2.8）。

Method according to CELSE

This method uses a rectangular excision of the affected segment of the lower lip. By means of a horizontal relaxing incision sublabially, two advancement flaps are created, which can be directly approximated. Two additional, auxiliary vertically arched incisions can be made in the region of the cheek. After approximation of the lower lip stumps, these can be closed secondarily (Fig. 2.8).

SERRE-MALGAIGNE方法（图2.9）

下唇再造的切口从嘴角横向两侧延伸，同时另外创建两条起自下唇缺损下缘同样向两侧延伸的平行切口。2个或所有4个切口贯穿整个脸颊皮肤肌肉和黏膜肌肉厚度，并到达咬肌前部边缘。为了更好地加强此经典推进皮瓣的弹性，PAYAN（1837）在内部黏膜皮瓣增加了垂直横向切口。RAEIS（1874）又做了进一步改进，建议在外部皮肤创建垂直切口。与之相反，SZYMAMOWSKI建议创建凹形切口皮瓣式样。GRANT建议通过将切口沿下颌下缘向下至舌骨，做1个梯形瓣（图2.9）。

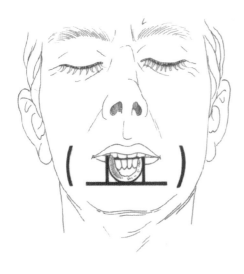

图2.8　CELSE方法

Fig. 2.8　Method according to CELSE

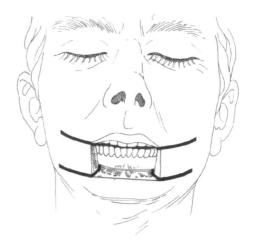

图2.9　SERRE-MALGAIGNE方法

Fig. 2.9　Method according to SERRE-MALGAIGNE

Method according to SERRE-MALGAIGNE (Fig. 2.9)

The incisions for lower lip reconstruction run horizontally from the corner of the mouth in a lateral direction. In addition, two parallel incisions are made, also laterally, beginning from the lower margin of the defect. Both or all four incisions are made through the full thickness of cutaneous muscle of the cheek and mucosa through to the anterior side of the masseter muscle. To improve elasticity of this classic advancement flap, PAYAN (1837) performs a lateral vertical incision in the inner mucosa flap. In another modification, REAIS (1874) recommends a vertical incision of the outer skin, while SZYMANOWSKI recommends a concave incision of the flap pedicle and GRANT recommends creating the flap in a trapeze shape by shifting the incision along the jawline and caudally towards the hyoid region (Fig. 2.9).

GROSS方法（图2.10）

这个方法是SERRE-MALGAIGNE方法的演变。它包括了另外两个在颏部位垂直的切口，从而实现了两个横向和一个纵向的肌皮瓣的推进（图2.10）。

Method according to GROSS (Fig. 2.10)

This method shows a variation of the method according to SERRE-MALGAIGNE. Here, two additional vertical incisions are made in the mental region. This allows the advancement of two lateral horizontal myocutaneous flaps and one vertical one (Fig. 2.10).

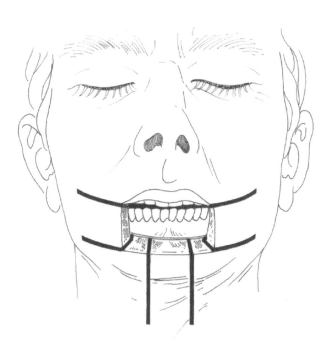

图2.10 GROSS方法

Fig. 2.10 Method according to GROSS

CHOPART方法（抽屉法）

在完全切除下唇后，创建两条纵向切口。切口从皮肤肌肉缺损处向下延伸到颏部（图2.11-1）。此松弛切口延伸至舌骨。将这个传统的推进皮瓣向颅侧推进。在下唇再造高度将剩余的前庭黏膜和皮肤缝合（图2.11-2）。

Method according to CHOPART (so-called "drawer method")

Following full excision of the lower lip, two vertical incisions are made, which lengthen the myocutaneous defect up to the chin (Fig. 2.11-1). This relaxing incision continues to the hyoid. A classic advancement flap is then shifted in a cranial direction. The remaining mucosa of the vestibule is sutured to the skin, level with the reconstructed lower lip (Fig. 2.11-2).

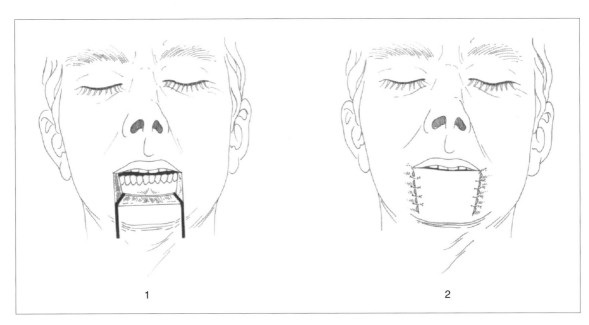

图2.11　CHOPART方法

Fig. 2.11　Method according to CHOPART

SZYMANOWSKI-CHOPART改良法

SZYMANOWSKI根据CHOPART方法进行了改进。通过创建一条位于切除创口尾部边缘的水平切口和两条尾端逼近的辅助切口形成一块颏皮瓣，宽度大于皮肤缺损。该皮瓣向颅侧的移动可实现下唇的"向前凸出"效果（图2.12）。

SZYMANOWSKI modified method according to CHOPART

SYZMANOWSKI modified the method according to CHOPART. Here, a chin flap is constructed by means of a horizontal incision in the area of the caudal resection edge as well as two converging auxiliary incisions. The chin flap is wider than the skin defect. To enable a "pouting" effect of the lower lip, this flap is advanced cranially (Fig. 2.12).

ALIQUIE方法（1885）

在CHOPART方法基础上进行改进。为了创建用于下唇外侧构造重建的肌皮瓣，在颊部两侧制作一块长方形黏膜皮瓣转90°并向内侧中央移植替代唇红（图2.13）。

Method according to ALQUIE (1885)

This is a modification of the method according to CHOPART. In addition to the construction of the myocutaneous flap used to reconstruct the exterior lower lip, a rectangular mucosal flap is made ambilaterally in the cheek area, which, after transposition by 90° medially replaces the lip vermilion (Fig. 2.13).

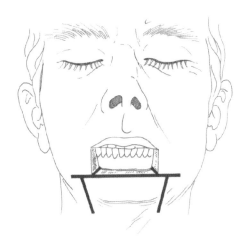

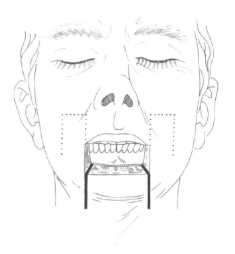

图2.12　SZYMANOWSKI–CHOPART改良法

Fig. 2.12　Method according to SZYMANOWSKI–CHOPART

图2.13　ALQUIE方法

Fig. 2.13　Method according to ALQUIE

ZEISS方法

这是CHOPART方法的另一种变化（图2.14）。这种改进的意义在于通过颏部区域的推进皮瓣的裤形切口，来避免由于瘢痕造成的再造下唇的下降。

Method according to ZEISS

This is yet another variation of Chopart's method (Fig. 2.14). The aim of this modification is to prevent sagging of the reconstructed lower lip caused by the scar. This is achieved with the aid of a "trouser-shaped" incision in the advancement flaps from the mental region.

SZYMANOWSKI方法

根据同ZEISS相同的原理，作者运用两条颏下部的向内凹陷的弧形皮瓣。SZYMANWSKI认为，通过这两个弧形切口可以完成下唇–颏部的整形再造。术后由于瘢痕原因造成的推进皮瓣向尾部偏移的情况可以降至最小（图2.15）。

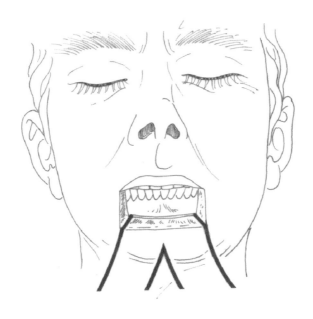

图2.14 ZEISS方法

Fig. 2.14 Method according to ZEISS

Method according to SZYMANOWSKI

In accordance with the principle described in the ZEISS method, this author uses two curved flaps from the submental region. These flaps have an inwardly concave form. In Szymanowski's opinion this curved incision enabled a plastic reconstruction of the lower lip and chin region. The aim was to avoid postoperative caudal shifting of the advancement flaps caused by the scar (Fig. 2.15).

其他SZYMANOWSKI改进方法

如图2.16所示，SZYMANOWSKI方法的又一种改进允许在口角部位切除两个三角形皮瓣。在下唇缺损下行至颏下部位创建一个V形切口后，会在两边口角切除一个三角形（图2.16）。通过这两个所创建的位于两侧正中的皮瓣向颅侧位移实现了下唇的再造。唇红由仍然存在的前庭黏膜构成。

Further modification of the method according to SZYMANOWSKI

One modification of the method shown in Fig. 2.16 allows for the excision of two triangular flaps from the region of the commissure of the mouth. First, a V-shaped incision is made from the lower lip defect running caudally to the submental region (Fig. 2.16). Then, two triangles are excised in the region of the labial commissures. Shifting each of the thus-formed paramedian skin flaps cranially results in reconstruction of the lower lip. The persisting vestibular mucosa is used to form the red lip.

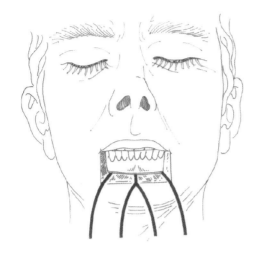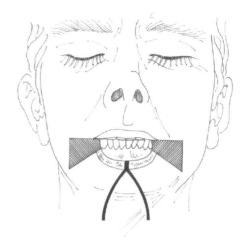

图2.15　SZYMANOWSKI方法

Fig. 2.15　Method according to SZYMANOWSKI

图2.16　SZYMANOWSKI改进方法

Fig. 2.16　Modification of the method
according to SZYMANOWSKI

通过外侧三角形推进皮瓣实现下唇再造

下唇局部损伤的再造，可以通过嘴角向颊部的水平方向松弛切口实现。通过这一切口可以建立一个三角形皮瓣，向中间旋转（图2.17）。由于皮瓣基部较大的宽度，弹性受到限制，从而只能可以实现下唇小范围缺损的修补。

Lower lip reconstruction by means of triangular lateral advancement flap

Reconstruction of a partial defect of the lower lip is made possible by performing a horizontal relaxing incision through the commissure of the mouth in the direction of the cheek. The result is a triangular flap, which is rotated medially (Fig. 2.17). Because the base of flap is considerably wide, elasticity is restricted. This type of defect coverage is therefore feasible only if loss of lower lip is minimal.

LISFRANC方法（1829）

此方法结合了伴有v形缺损的下唇向舌骨方向垂直的切口和两条水平穿过嘴角至颊部的向上微微凸的切口。切口的终点位于咬肌前缘，通过松动这两块三角形皮瓣来完成内侧旋转（图2.18）。

Method according to LISFRANC (1829)

This method combines a vertical incision from the V-shaped lower lip defect towards the hyoid, and two horizontal incisions through the commissure of the mouth into the cheek region. The horizontal incisions are slightly convex upwardly. The end of the incision is situated on the anterior margin of the masseter muscle. Both of the triangular flaps are mobilized and then medially rotated (Fig. 2.18).

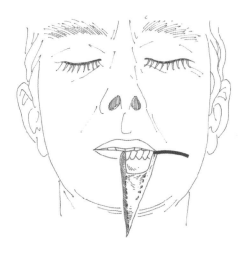 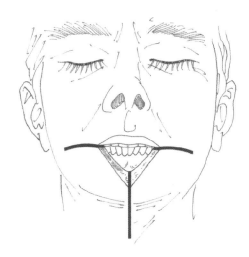

图2.17　外侧三角形推进皮瓣方法

Fig. 2.17　Triangular lateral advancement flap

图2.18　LISFRANC方法

Fig. 2.18　Method according to LISFRANC

MALGAIGNE方法（1834）

此方法基本上与LISFRANC方法有相同的再造思路。只是放弃了垂直方向的中间切口（图2.19）。相同的方法由BONNET在1838年也进行过描述。

Method according to MALGAIGNE (1834)

This method is based on the same reconstructive idea as that of the LISFRANC method. Only this method does not use the vertical, median incision (Fig. 2.19). The same procedure was described by BONNET in 1838.

SEDILLOT方法（1856）

此方法也是通过推进两块颊部的三角形皮瓣来再造下唇V形缺损的。作一个2cm辅助切口，该切口在唇红缘向上内行，与上唇相切，来实现上唇侧部的向下旋转，从而达到再造修补下唇（图2.20）。这种方法同样在1889年被MORESTIN和SILBERBERG所采用。

Method according to SEDILLOT (1856)

This method, too, advances two triangular flaps from the cheek area to reconstruct a V-shaped defect of the lower lip. A supplementary auxiliary incision is made; it is 2 cm in length and runs tangent to the upper lip cranio-medially in the vicinity of the vermilion. This auxiliary incision permits rotation of the lateral upper-lip segment downwards in order to reconstruct the lip (Fig. 2.20). This method was also used by MORESTIN and SILBERBERG in 1889.

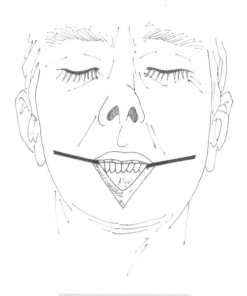

图2.19 MALGAIGNE方法

Fig. 2.19 Method according to MALGAIGNE

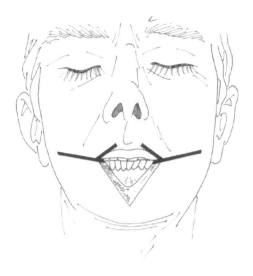

图2.20 SEDILLOT方法

Fig. 2.20 Method according to SEDILLOT

DIEFFENBACH方法

在下唇进行V形切除后，在嘴角两侧创建两条从嘴角至鼻唇沟中部的辅助切口。再通过一条额外的鼻唇沟延长线至颏部的切口可以创建两块顶端几乎接触的小三角形皮瓣。这种方法可以重建出两侧圆形的嘴角（图2.21）。

Method according to DIEFFENBACH

After V-shaped excision of the lower lip, two lateral auxiliary incisions are made which run from the commissure of the mouth to the medial nasolabial region. An additional incision made in continuation of

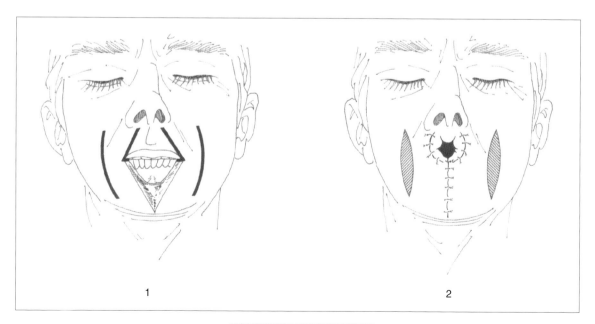

图2.21 DIEFFENBACH方法

Fig. 2.21 Method according to DIEFFENBACH

the nasolabial groove and running to the chin area permits the formation of two smaller triangular flaps, the angles of which can be directly approximated. The result is a bilaterally rounded commissure of the mouth (Fig. 2.21).

DESGRANGE方法（1853/1854）

在下唇V形切除后，伤口直接缝合。为了再造口裂，在嘴角高度两侧颊部水平各开一条约2.5cm长贯穿切口（A-B）。然后再作一条45°颅向，1.5cm长切口（B-C）。通过连接C点和A点在两侧各切除一个三角形黏膜肌皮瓣。A-C和B-C伤口边缘再直接缝合。由此口裂被拉伸并呈流线型。通过将口腔黏膜沿A-B切口向外翻转最终实现再造下唇红（图2.22）。

Method according to DESGRANGE (1853/1854)

Following V-shaped excision of the lower lip, the wound margins are directly approximated. In order to reconstruct the oral opening, a vertical cut 2.5 cm in length is made through the full thickness of the cheek area bilaterally and level with the commissure of the mouth (A-B). A further incision (B-C) 1.5cm, long is made at a 45° angle cranially. By joining the points C and A, a triangle consisting of cutaneous muscle and mucosa is excised. The wound margins A-C and B-C are then approximated by means of a direct suture. The oral opening is thus broadened and the upper lip tightened. Outward rotation of the mucosa along the line A-B allows for reconstruction of the lower lip vermilion (Fig. 2.22).

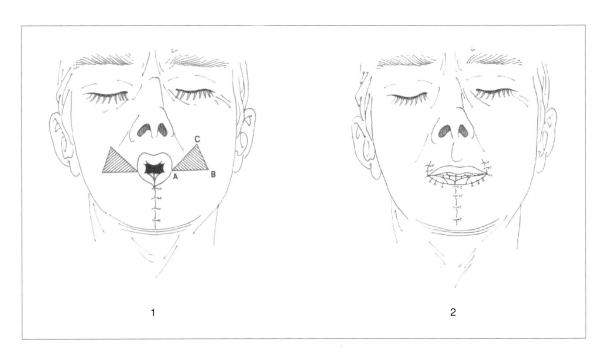

图2.22　DESGRANGE方法

Fig. 2.22　Method according to DESGRANGE

ROUX方法

根据此方法，会将下唇肿瘤通过非对称V形切口切除。V形短端向颈部延长并将创建侧部的三角形皮瓣颅侧上行推进（图2.23）。

Method according to ROUX

This method removes the lower lip tumor by means of an asymmetric V-shaped excision. The shorter side of the asymmetric V is lengthened in a cervical direction and the resulting lateral triangular flap is advanced in a cranial direction (Fig. 2.23).

SZYMANOWSKI方法

根据SZYMANOWSKI的改进，辅助切口改为向外下部方向的小波浪形。由此达到更好的口-颏部区域的再造修复效果（图2.24）。

Method according to SZYMANOWSKI

In a modification of SZYMANOWSKI's, the auxiliary incision follows a slightly undulated course in a lateral caudal direction. This form permits a better reconstruction of the mouth and chin regions (Fig. 2.24).

BEAU方法（1869）

此方法中运用了凹形切口来切除肿瘤，在凹形切口的最低点向下颌下部方向创建两条内凹形辅助切口（图2.25-1）。松动两侧皮瓣，并将其向上推进。再造修复后的最终效果不再有组织丢失（图2.25-2）。这种方法不会产生额外的结缔组织损失。

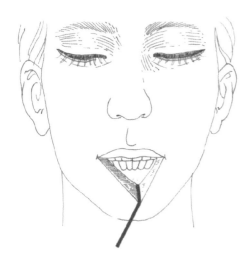

图2.23 ROUX方法

Fig. 2.23 Method according to ROUX

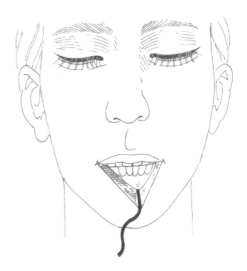

图2.24 SZYMANOWSKI方法

Fig. 2.24 Method according to SZYMANOWKSI

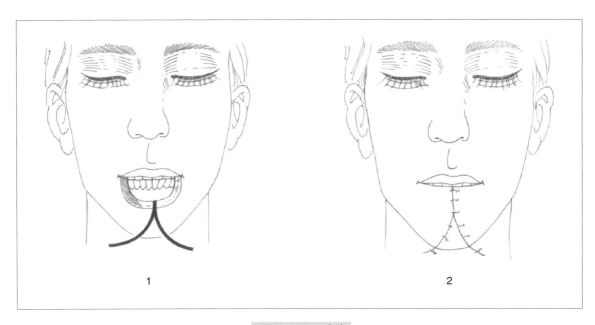

图2.25 BEAU方法

Fig. 2.25   Method according to BEAU

Method according to BEAU (1869)

Here, tumor excision is carried out via a concave resection of the lower lip. Beginning from the lowest point of the concave resection, two auxiliary incisions are developed which run in an outwardly concave line up to the submandibular area (Fig. 2.25-1). These lateral flaps are then mobilized and shifted in a cranial direction. Fig. 2.25-2 shows the final result after reconstruction of the lip. No further tissue loss occurs.

BLASIUS可能是SZYMANOWSKI之后第一个描述了这一方法的人。

According to SZYMANOWSKI, the first author to describe this method seems to have been BLASIUS.

ERICHSEN方法

在下唇完全切除后，为实现下唇的再造修复，将会在两侧水平方向切除一个四边形肌皮瓣，在内侧中间切除一个三角形肌皮瓣。所形成的两侧咬肌区的三角形皮瓣最终向上推进并缝合在一起。此方法的缺点在于舍弃了口部两侧和颏下区的健康的结缔组织（图2.26）。

Method according to ERICHSEN

Following total resection of the lower lip, two lateral, horizontal, rectangular flaps and one triangular median cutaneous muscle excision are developed in order to carry out reconstruction. Each of the two resulting triangular flaps from the lateral mental region are subsequently shifted in an upward direction and joined/adapted with a suture. The downfall of this method is that healthy tissue from the lateral oral and submental regions must be sacrificed (Fig. 2.26).

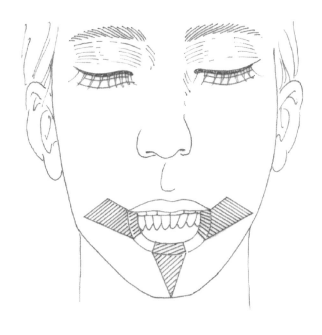

图2.26　ERICHSEN方法

Fig. 2.26　Method according to ERICHSEN

JOHANSON方法

JOHANSON在1884年描述了该技术。显示了一种次全下唇缺损的整形术。图2.27-1描述了下唇肿瘤切除的切口形状，三角阶梯状辅助切口向两侧向下延伸和在两边下颌下缘切除的Burrow三角形。这些切口贯穿所有下唇和脸颊组织层。

Method according to JOHANSON

JOHANSON described this technique in 1884. The indication is a subtotal defect plasty of the lower lip. Fig. 2.27-1 shows development of an incision to excise a lower lip tumor. It also shows the development of a triangular, lateral caudal auxiliary incision and the removal of bilateral Burrow's triangles at the edge of the mandible. The incision is carried out through all thicknesses of the lower lip and cheek.

图2.27-2是肿瘤切除后的情况和梯形辅助切口。

Fig2.27-2 illustrates the situation following tumor excision and shows the staircase-shaped auxiliary incision.

图2.27-3描述了缝合后的效果。

Fig2.27-3 shows the final result.

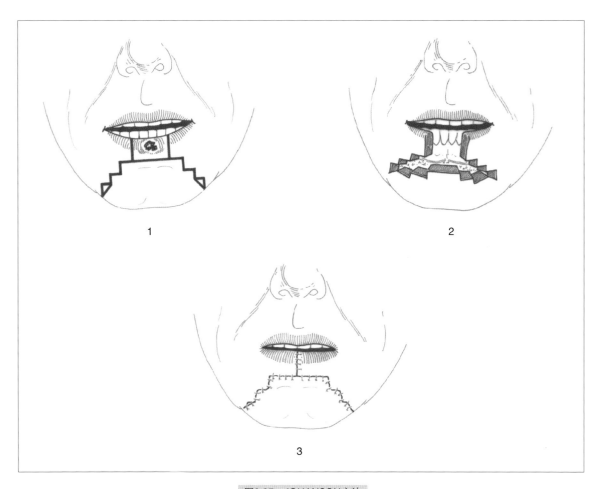

1

2

3

图2.27　JOHANSON方法

Fig. 2.27　Method according to JOHANSON

GOLDSTEIN方法

　　针对仅仅唇红缺损的情况，GOLDSTEIN在1983年描述了用扩张肌皮组织唇红皮瓣来修复红唇缺失。适用病情扩展到下唇红缺损小于50%，如在唇红部位受到损伤、烧伤或者癌症前期在唇红区域出现病变。图2.28-1表示了剩余的下唇红的推进。虚线表示唇红皮瓣切口的走向。图2.28-2是掀起的含有动脉的唇红皮瓣。唇红皮瓣横切面的基部呈反V字形。通过伸展和延长唇红皮瓣达到覆盖患处的目的（图2.28-3）。图2.28-4显示了重建后的最终效果。

Method according to GOLDSTEIN

In 1983, GOLDSTEIN described the use of a myocutaneous tissue-expanding vermilion flap for primary reconstruction where a vermilion-only defect is present. This method is indicated to bridge a loss of less than 50% of the lower lip vermilion, incurred by injuries and burn traumas or precancerous changes in the red lip area. Fig. 2.28-1 outlines shifting of the remaining lower lip vermilion. The dotted line shows the continuous incision of the vermilion flap, Fig. 2.28-2 shows the raised arterialized myocutaneous vermilion flap. The base of the cross-section of the lip vermilion flap has an inverted V-shape. Stretching or elongating the vermilion flap permits closure of the defect (Fig. 2.28-3). Fig. 2.28-4 illustrates the end result after reconstruction.

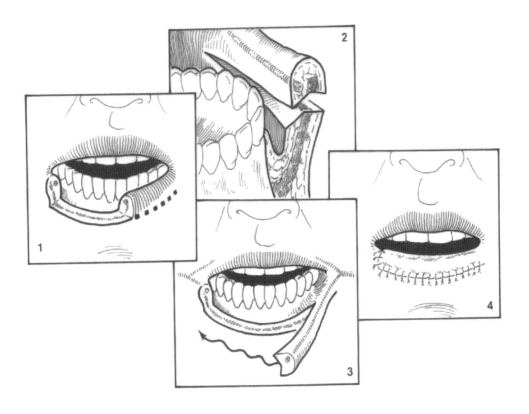

图2.28 GOLDSTEIN方法

Fig. 2.28 Method according to GOLDSTEIN

BERNARD方法

　　BERNARD的方法是通过横向推进皮瓣来实现全下唇缺损的再造。图2.29-1展示了贯穿所有下唇组织层的肿瘤楔形切口。鼻旁各切除一个几乎为等腰三角形，其底部位于口裂处。从中获取黏膜为下唇红再造之用。图2.29-2描述了通过外下的两瓣推进，展示皮瓣最后缝合的效果。唇红的再造是通过转移来自鼻旁Burrow氏三角形切除区域的黏膜瓣来完成的。

Method according to BERNARD

With the method according to BERNARD (1853) reconstruction of a total lower lip defect can be achieved by means of lateral advancement flaps. Fig. 2.29-1 demonstrates wedge-shaped excision of the lower lip tumor through all thicknesses of the lower lip. Paranasally, on both sides, two nearly equilateral triangles are excised. Their bases are in continuation with the commissure line. The mucosa is retained; it serves to reconstruct the lower lip vermilion. The final result after approximation of both advancement flaps from a lateral caudal direction is shown in Fig. 2.29-2 Reconstruction of the red lip was achieved by transposing the mucosal flaps from the region of the excised paranasal Burrow's triangles.

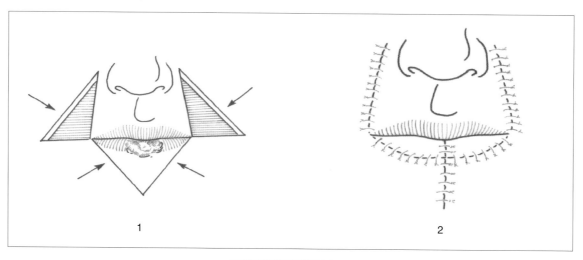

图2.29　BERNARD方法

Fig. 2.29　Method according to BERNARD

根据BERNARD方法改进的FRIES方法（1）

FRIES（1973）改进了BERNARD的方法，通过横向推进皮瓣实现下唇局部缺损的修复。图2.30-1展示了一个贯穿所有组织层的用以切除下唇肿瘤的心形切口。口裂两侧创建一条稍稍向上的辅助切口，该切口也贯穿了所有的脸颊皮肤层。切口经过颊黏膜处要高于经过皮肤，以便通过向外翻转黏膜来实现唇红的再造修复。图2.30-2显示了下唇重建的最后状态。

Modification to BERNARD method according to FRIES (1)

FRIES (1973) modified the BERNARD method for reconstruction of subtotal lower lip defects by means of lateral advancement flaps. Fig. 2.30-1 demonstrates removal of a lower lip tumor by means of a heart-shaped excision carried out through the full thickness of the lower lip. An auxiliary excision in

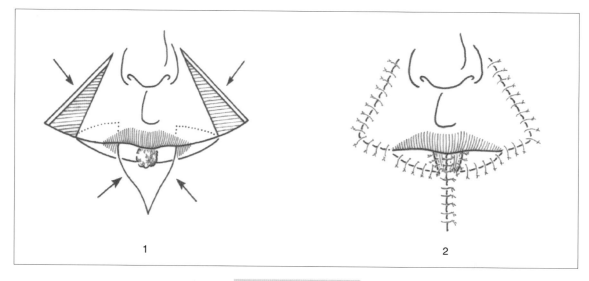

图2.30　FRIES方法（1）

Fig. 2.30　Method according to FRIES（1）

continuation of the commissure line and running in a slightly cranial direction through all thicknesses of the cheek is developed bilaterally. The incision through the buccal mucosa is developed on a higher level than that one crossing the dermis; this enables reconstruction of the red lip by means of outwardly rotated mucosa. The final result after lower lip reconstruction is shown in Fig. 2.30-2.

在推进两侧面颊皮瓣后，下唇患处的切口边缘将直接缝合，唇红通过颊黏膜再造修复。鼻旁处等腰三角形的愈合避免了鼻唇沟附近的软组织凸起。

After advancement of the lateral buccal flaps, the excision edges of the lower lip defect are directly approximated. The red lip is reconstructed by means of buccal mucosa. Adaptation of the equilateral sides of the paranasal triangles prevents the formation of raised soft tissue in the nasolabial region.

FRIES方法（2）

FRIES在1973年同样描述了下唇外侧缺损再造的一种方法。

Method according to FRIES (2)

In 1973, FRIES also described a method for reconstructing lateral lower lip defects.

图2.31-1显示了用以切除位于下唇单侧的下唇肿瘤的心形切口和在鼻唇沟处切除的Burrow氏三角形。此处切口经过黏膜处也是高于水平方向切除区皮肤。向内侧推进皮瓣后对位缝合，对应唇红的一块皮肤会除去。保留的黏膜向外翻转，由此通过侧面面颊区的黏膜再造了唇红。

Fig. 2.31-1 shows heart-shaped development of an incision for removal of a laterally situated lower lip tumor and excision of a Burrow's triangle in the nasolabial region. Here, too, the incision line runs higher in the mucosal area than the horizontal relaxing incision in the dermis. After medial transposition of advancement flaps and adaptation of the wound edges, a strip of skin is removed which corresponds in size and shape to the red lip. The preserved mucosa is rotated outwardly, thus reconstructing the red lip from the mucosa of the lateral buccal region.

图2.31-2显示了面颊皮瓣向内侧旋转后的最终状态。

Fig. 2.31-2 shows the final state after medial rotation of the caudal buccal flap.

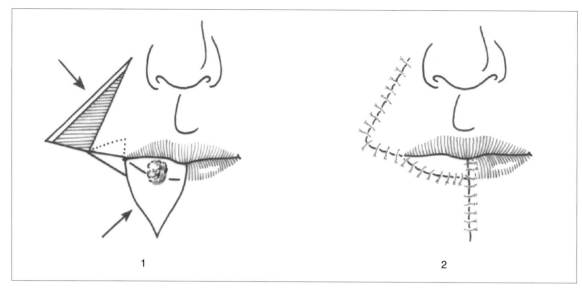

图2.31　FRIES方法（2）

Fig. 2.31　Method according to FRIES（2）

FRIES方法（3）

此方法的适应证为下唇矩形缺损。

Method according to FRIES (3)

This technique is indicated for rectangular defects of the lower lip.

图2.32-1表示了下唇肿瘤，其通过一矩形切口贯穿所有皮肤组织层被切除。辅助切口水平向经嘴角两侧连合部向颏下延伸。在颏下，下颌下和鼻唇沟区各切除两块等腰Burrow氏三角形皮瓣。

Fig. 2.32-1 demonstrates removal of a lower lip tumor by means of a rectangular excision through all thicknesses of the lower lip. Bilateral auxiliary incisions run horizontally through the commissure submentally. Here, too, two equilateral Burrow's triangles are excised in the submental or submandibular and in the nasolabial regions.

相对于BERNARD-FRIES方法，此方法在切除了下唇后，在缺损边缘下部向侧面下部额外创建了一条松弛切口。下颌下所切除的两块等腰三角形可以防止下颌下的皮肤凸起。

This method is like that of BERNARD-FRIES, only in addition, a relaxing excision is made after lower lip resection, which runs from the caudal defect margin in a lateral caudal direction. Submandibular excision of two equilateral triangles precludes excessive rising of the dermis in the submandibular region.

图2.32-2显示了用颊黏膜修复唇红区的效果。

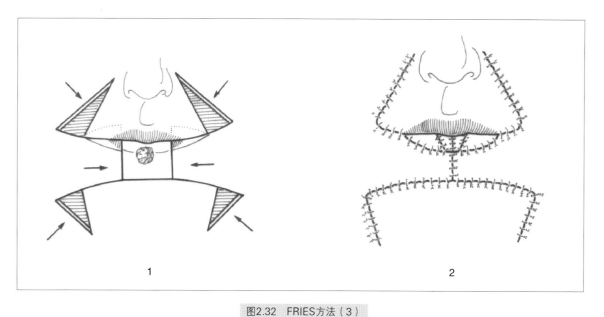

图2.32 FRIES方法（3）

Fig. 2.32 Method according to FRIES（3）

Fig. 2.32-2 shows the result after approximation of the advancement flaps and reconstruction of the red lip using buccal mucosa.

BERNARD氏唇整形的肌整形改良

最先由FREEMAN在1958年提出。适用范围为下唇缺损大于30%的下唇再造修复。图2.33-1显示了肿瘤切除后的状态。两侧嘴角Burrow氏三角形切除，并保留脸颊黏膜。下唇部位的整形能够通过两条两侧水平的切口实现。唇红两侧边打点的区域表示要切除的三角形皮瓣。将其切除后，伤口边缘同保留的口腔黏膜相缝合来实现下唇的再造（图2.33-2）。

Myoplastic modification of BERNARD's lip plastic surgery

This technique was first described in the year 1958 by FREEMAN. The method is indicated for reconstruction of a lower lip defect involving over 30% of the lower lip. Fig. 2.33-1 shows the appearance after tumor excision. In addition, it shows bilaterally excised Burrows's triangles in the region of the oral commissure, whereby the buccal mucosa is preserved. Advancement plastic surgery in the region of the lower lip is performed by means of two lateral and horizontal incisions. The stippled area on both sides lateral to the lower lip vermilion shows the dermal triangle which will be excised. After removal of the triangles, the wound edges are sutured to the preserved oral mucosa, thereby reconstructing the lower lip (Fig. 2.33-2).

图2.33-3显示了修复后的唇红和唇白间的皮肤缝合后的状态。图2.33-4显示了最终的结果。

Fig. 2.33-3 shows the appearance after performance of the dermal sutures between the reconstructed red lip and the white lip. Fig. 2.33-4 shows the end result.

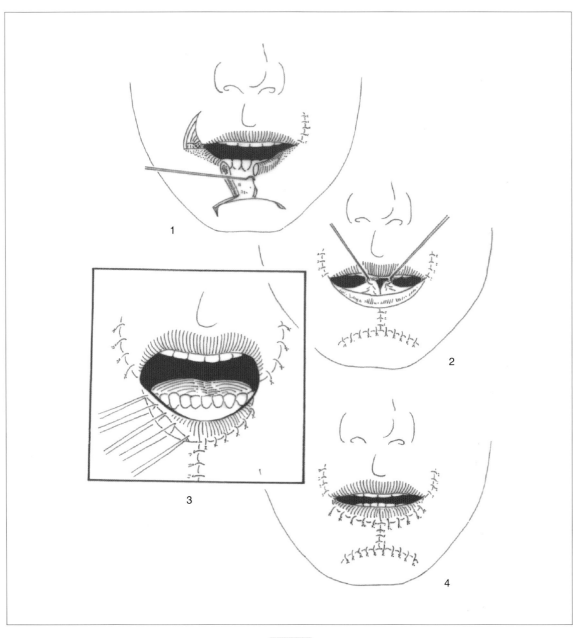

图2.33

Fig. 2.33

图2.34提供了关于嘴角区域三层修复的详细信息。

Fig. 2.34 show the details of three-layered reconstruction in the oral commissure.

图2.34显示了切除嘴角外侧Burrow氏三角形皮瓣后的状态。鼻唇沟区域皮肤已经切除。口轮匝肌被保护起来。最终完成面颊黏膜与口轮匝肌黏膜剥离（图2.34-2）。然后口轮匝肌用圆形可吸收线结扎，从而形成侧面的偏移。保留的黏膜将用于之后的唇红再造（图2.34-3）。

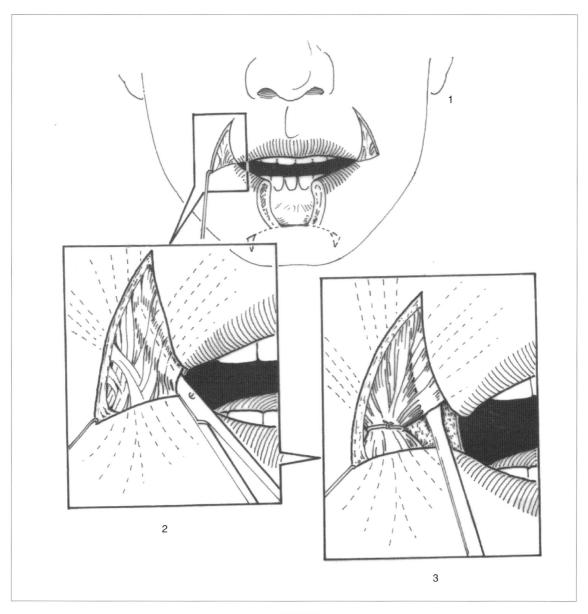

图2.34

Fig. 2.34

Fig. 2.34-1 shows the appearance after excision of the Burrow's triangle situated laterally to the oral commissure. The skin in the nasolabial region has already been removed. The orbicularis oris muscle remains intact. Subsequently, the buccal mucosa is submucosally detached from the orbicularis oris muscle (Fig. 2.34-2). Then, the orbicular muscle is gathered by means of a circular absorbable suture, whereby it is shifted in a lateral direction. The preserved mucosa is used for subsequent reconstruction of the red lip (Fig. 2.34-3).

改良的BERNARD氏手术

适应证为下唇缺损小于2/3范围。图2.35-1显示了切除一较宽下唇肿瘤的切口线和在口裂两侧创建的两块Burrow氏三角形。通过切除这两块Burrow氏三角形皮瓣可以创建面颊-唇-推进皮瓣，同时可避免出现"猫耳"。

Modified BERNARD Operation

This method is indicated when the lower lip defect involves less than two thirds of the width of the lower lip. Fig. 2.35-1 shows the line of incision for excision of a broad lower lip tumor and the creation of two Burrow's triangles laterally to the oral commissure on both sides. The excision of these Burrow's triangles enables the formation of a cheek-lip-advancement flap without "dog-ear or pig-ear".

Burrow氏三角区的口腔黏膜将被保留，用以修复转移面颊−下唇−肌皮瓣部分后所形成的唇部黏膜缺损。Burrow氏三角形的基部为圆弧形。最终状态可见图2.35−2。

The oral mucosa in the region of the Burrow's triangles is meticulously preserved, so that the labial mucosal defect which results after advancement of the cheek-lower lip-myocutaneous segments can be reconstructed. The base of the Burrow's triangles is slightly curved. The end result is shown in Fig. 2.35-2.

BERNARD−TYP手术

这种手术技术是根据BERNARD氏方法改良而来。适应证为全下唇缺损并必须额外切除下唇−颏下区皮肤的情况。再造通过两侧推进皮瓣完成。此方法可实现功能满意的下唇再造，但是给予患者造成典型的无表情下唇形状。

BERNARD-Type Operation

This operative technique is a modification of the operation according to BERNARD. It is indicated for defects of the entire lower lip and when, in addition, it is necessary to remove the skin of the lower lip chin area. Reconstruction is carried out by means of advancing flaps from a lateral direction. This method creates

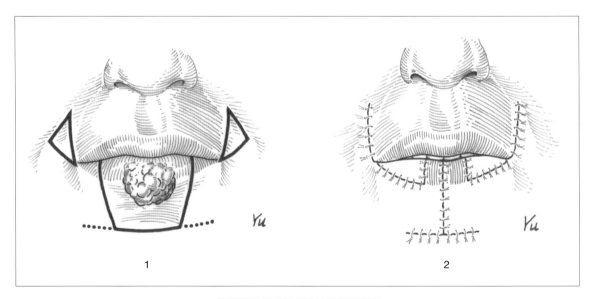

图2.35　改良的BERNARD氏手术

Fig. 2.35　Modified BERNARD Operation

a functionally satisfactory reconstruction of the lower lip, however, it leaves the patient with a typically expressionless lower lip form.

图2.36-1显示了切除大肿物的切口线和在口角旁两个Burrow氏三角形的切口线。

Fig. 2.36-1 shows the line of incision for the excision of a broad tumor and two Burrow's triangles laterally from the oral commissure.

图2.36-2中描绘了背向延伸的切口边缘，其尾部两侧延伸至下颌下区域并成楔形基底结束。三角形底部对应下唇缺损范围的一半。三角形定点结束于鼻唇沟延长线方向。

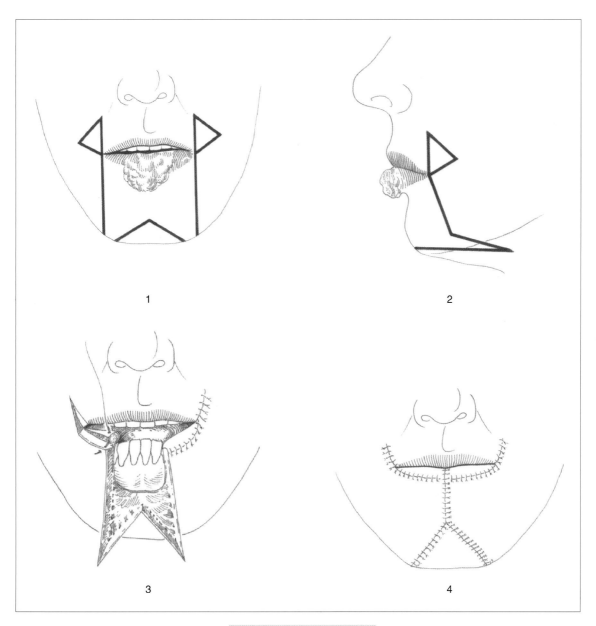

图2.36　BERNARD-TYP手术

Fig. 2.36　BERNARD-Type Operation

Fig. 2.36-2 shows the borders of the excision, which reaches dorsally, and which runs in a lateral caudal direction in the submandibular region and ends in a wedge-formed base. The base of each triangle corresponds to one half of the extension of the defect of the lower lip. The corners of the triangles end in a continuation of the nasolabial groove.

如图2.36-3所示，贯穿所有下唇组织层和颏部肌肉组织的切口和在切除Burrow氏三角时保留面颊黏膜，并以其修复唇红。下唇再造后的最终状态见图2.36-4。

The excision is performed through all thicknesses of the lower lip and chin muscle as shown in Fig. 2.36-3. During excision of the Burrow's triangles, the mucosa of the cheek is preserved and used to reconstruct the red lip. The end result after lower lip reconstruction can be seen in Fig. 2.36-4.

DIEFFENBACH方法（1845—1848）

这种方法适用于V形下唇全部缺损。通过在口裂延长线方向上创建的辅助切口和竖直的松弛切口可以在腮腺区形成两块矩形颊皮瓣，其将可以向中间平移。

Method according to DIEFFENBACH (1845-1848)

This method is indicated for full, V-shaped lower lip defects. After creation of an auxiliary incision in continuation of the oral commissure and of a vertical relaxing incision, two rectangular buccal flaps can be formed in the parotid region. These flaps are transposed medially.

切口起于嘴角两侧并向耳屏方向延伸，止于耳屏前大约1.5cm处。同时需避开咬肌筋膜和腮腺筋膜。保护颊黏膜。两侧动脉和静脉须结扎。在耳屏前1.5cm处，创建一条垂直向下经过下颌边缘的切口。将周围切开的颊软组织瓣从咬肌和深入腮腺的筋膜分离。Enoral在口内皮肤切口上方1cm处切开黏膜（虚线，图2.37-1）并最终向外旋转，用于再造唇红。为了能够覆盖口内带有黏膜的创面，必须松动下颌黏骨膜瓣，然后向内侧移动颊瓣，并在中线使用间断缝合（图2.37-2）。

The incision line runs bilaterally from the oral commissure in the direction of the tragus and ends approximately 1.5 cm. before it reaches the tragus. The fascia of the masseter muscle and of the parotid must not be opened. The mucosa of the cheek is primarily preserved. The facial artery and vein are ligated bilaterally. At a distance of 1.5 cm. from the tragus a vertical incision is made downwards which extends beyond the border of the lower jaw. The circumcised buccal soft tissue flap is dissected off of the masseter and the fascia which cuts into the parotid gland. Intraorally, the mucosa is circumcised horizontally 1 cm above the skin incision (dotted line, Fig. 2.37-1) and subsequently rotated outwards in order to reconstruct the red lip. The mucoperiosteum of the lower jaw must then be mobilized in order to be able to cover the oral wound surface with mucosa. Then, the buccal flaps are shifted medially and approximated in the midline with interrupted sutures (Fig. 2.37-2).

图2.37-3展示了下唇修复后的最终状态。

Fig. 2.37-3 now shows the end result of the reconstructed lower lip.

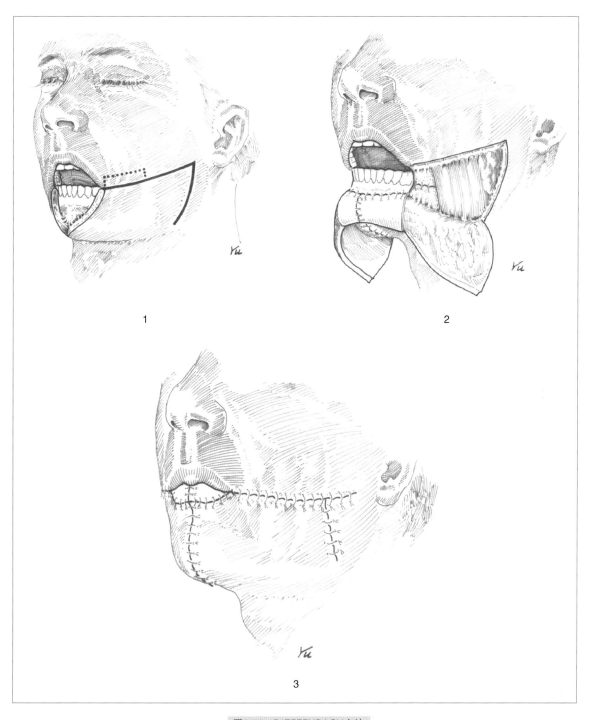

图2.37 DIEFFENBACH方法

Fig. 2.37 Method according to DIEFFENBACH

此方法的优点在于可以在再造下唇缺损的同时通过颊黏膜完成下唇红的修复。

The advantage of this method is that coverage of a total lower lip defect is possible. At the same time, the red lip can be restored using buccal mucosa.

缺点则是再造后的下唇的功能缺失和由于辅助切口延伸至腮腺区域而造成的广泛瘢痕。由于运动神经的大范围分离，使得再生和恢复极其缓慢。

The drawback of this method is a loss of function of the restored lower lip and extensive scar formation caused by auxiliary incisions reaching into the parotid region. Motor innervation is largely divided; this greatly delays regeneration.

图2.38描述了CONVERSE对此方法进行的改良。同时表明他运用了来自上唇的STEIN-KAZAJIAN皮瓣。

Fig. 2.38 shows a modification of this method according to CONVERSE and indicates the additional implementation of STEIN-KAZANJIAN flaps from the upper lip.

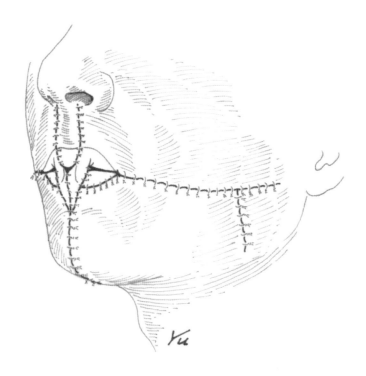

图2.38　CONVERSE方法

Fig. 2.38　Method according to CONVERSE

SCHUCHARDT方法

Schuchardt于1944年描述了一种运用推进皮瓣的下唇再造方法。此方法可运用于下唇中部缺损的再造。

Method according to SCHUCHARDT

In 1944 Schuchardt described an advancement plastic surgery technique for lower lip reconstruction. This method is indicated for defects in the middle lower lip region.

图2.39-1展示了下唇中部的缺损，以及所创建的向下弯曲的圆弧形切口线。在松弛切口的末端，颏下的颈部皮肤两侧各切除一块Burrow氏三角皮瓣。松动这两个皮瓣，并将其向内向上方旋转，然后间断缝合。图2.39-2显示了已闭合的左侧前庭黏膜。

Fig. 2.39-1 shows the medial defect of the lower lip and the planned, downwardly arched line of incision. At the end of the relaxing incision, a Burrow's triangle is excised from the skin of the throat submentally on each side. Each of the two lip stumps are then mobilized and rotated upwardly in a medial direction before they are approximated by means of interrupted sutures. Fig. 2.39-2 shows the sutured vestibular mucosa on the left side.

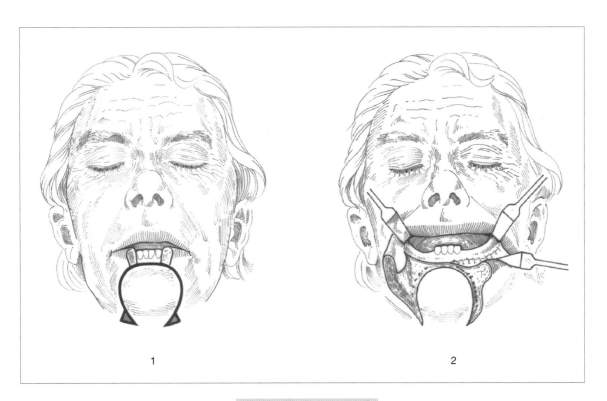

1

2

图2.39　SCHUCHARDT方法

Fig. 2.39　Method according to SCHUCHARDT

对于GRIMM方法改进的LUHR方法（1970）

此方法结合了BERNARD、BURROW、DIEFFENBACH和SCHUCHARDT各方法并同时配合运用颌下淋巴结群清除术切口线。

Modification of the GRIMM Method according to LUHR (1970)

This technique is a combination of the BERNARD, BURROW, DIEFFENBACH and SCHUCHARDT methods with an additional incision line for the dissection of the submandibular lymph node group.

图2.40-1展示了切口线路：在鼻唇区切除Burrow氏三角，环绕颏部直至下颌的弧形切口并延伸用于舌骨上淋巴结清除术。虚线描绘了黏膜区域的切口。

Fig. 2.40-1 shows the course of the incision: excision of Burrow's triangles in the nasolabial region, an arched incision around the region of the chin extending submentally, and the continuation of the incision for suprahyoid lymph node dissection. The dotted lines show the incision in the region of the mucosa.

图2.40-2展示了进行肿瘤切除、淋巴结清除术和两侧颊部平移皮瓣移动后的状态。所切开的黏膜皮瓣要大于肌皮瓣，并由此通过向外旋转多余的黏膜皮瓣来完成唇红的再造修复。

Fig. 2.40-2 shows the appearance after tumor excision, lymph node dissection and bilateral mobilization of the advancement flaps from the inferior buccal region. The mucosal flaps were made larger than the myocutaneous flaps in order to enable a reconstruction of the red lip by means of outward rotation of the excess mucosa.

图2.40-3展示了最终的状态。通过切除鼻唇沟侧的Burrow氏三角，可使脸颊部位的缺损无软组织扭曲而闭合。脸颊黏膜用来再造修复唇红。

Fig. 2.40-3 shows the final result. Excision of Burrow's triangles laterally to the nasolabial sulcus permits coverage of the cheek defect without heaping up of soft tissue. The buccal mucosa is used to reconstruct the red lower lip.

WEBSTER方法

1960年WEBSTER和其工作人员描述了另一种基于Bernard方法改进的方法，用于再造修复全下唇缺损。

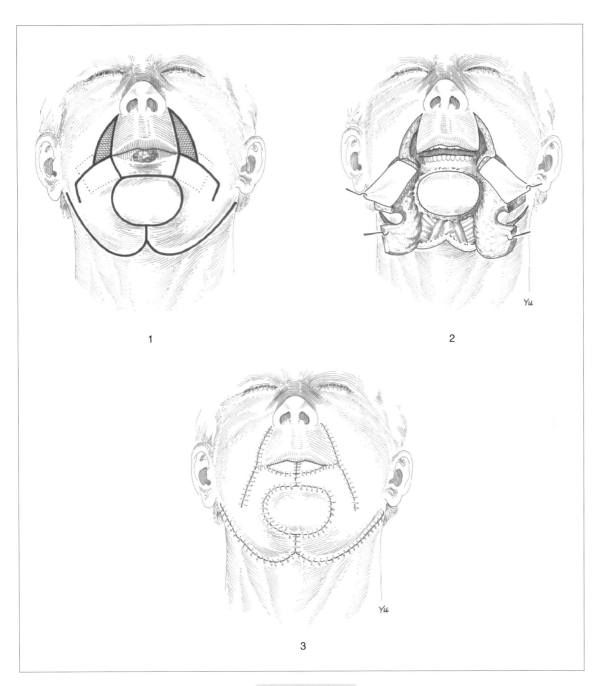

1

2

3

图2.40 LUHR方法

Fig. 2.40 Method according to LUHR

Method according to WEBSTER

In 1960, WEBSTER and associates described a further modification of the Bernard technique for reconstruction of a total lower lip defect.

图2.41-1展示了用于切除较宽的唇肿瘤及贯穿全层的辅助切口的切口线。两块软组织皮瓣及相连面颊软组织推进并直接缝合。这可通过事先切除的Burrow氏三角形或Imre氏半月形来实现。唇红则由相邻的面颊黏膜来再造。图2.41-2显示了最终状态。

Fig. 2.41-1 shows the incision line for excision of a broad lip tumor and the full-thickness auxiliary incisions. Both lip and buccal soft tissue stumps are mobilized and directly approximated. This is made possible by prior excision of Burrow's triangles or half moons according to Imre. The red lip is reconstructed from the adjacent buccal mucosa. Fig. 2.41-2 shows the final result.

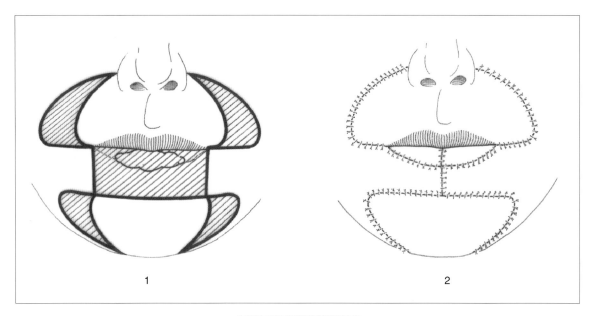

1　　　2

图2.41　WEBSTER方法

Fig. 2.41　Method according to WEBSTER

GRIMM方法（1966）

此方法也可用于全下唇缺损的再造。

Method according to GRIMM (1966)

This method, too, allows for reconstruction of a total lower lip defect.

图2.42-1描述了用于切除较宽的下唇癌的方形切口线，两侧鼻唇沟外侧的Burrow氏三角形位置以及两侧下颌额外的Burrow氏三角形。虚线表示了设计的黏膜切口，其高于肌皮瓣切口的位置。

Fig. 2.42-1 shows the square incision line carried out to excise a broad lower lip carcinoma. It also shows the creation of Burrow's triangles on both sides laterally to the nasolabial fold and submentally. The dotted lines show the planned mucosal incisions. These are situated on a higher level than the myocutaneous incision.

图2.42-2显示了切除肿瘤后的状态，作松弛切口和形成黏膜瓣，后者以后用于唇红再造。

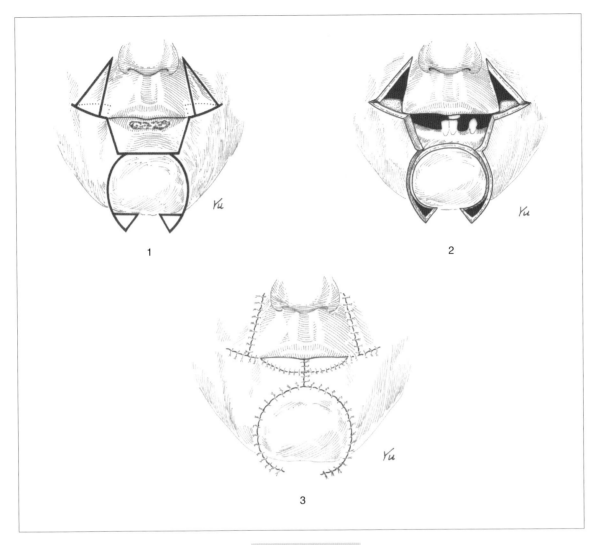

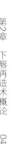

图2.42 GRIMM方法

Fig. 2.42 Method according to GRIMM

Fig. 2.42-2 shows the condition after tumor excision, creation of the relaxing incisions and formation of the mucosa flaps. The latter will later serve for reconstruction of the lip vermilion.

图2.42-3显示了最终状态。

Fig. 2.42-3 shows the end result.

3. 旋转皮瓣

ADELMANN方法

根据ADELMANN所描述的方法，运用同DIEFFENBACH技术一样，环切两个面颊皮瓣。不同之处在于切口将不穿过黏膜。所形成的面颊皮瓣也大于使用传统的DIEFFENBACH方法做的皮瓣一直扩展到咬肌区域。推进皮瓣至中线并直接缝合后，咬肌将被暴露（图2.43）。

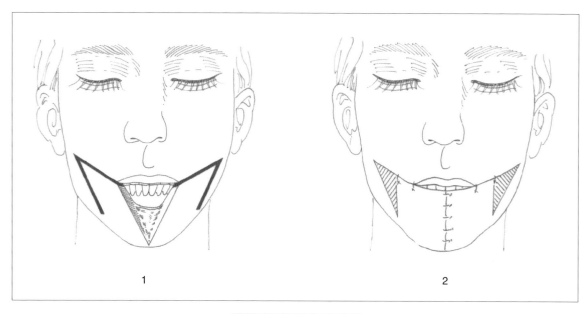

图2.43   ADELMANN方法

Fig. 2.43   Method according to ADELMANN

3. Rotational Flaps

Method according to ADELMANN

The method described by ADELMANN circumcises two buccal flaps, such as are described in the DIEFFENBACH technique. However, it differs in that the incisions do not traverse the mucosa. The created buccal flaps are larger in size than in the classical method according to DIEFFENBACH and they extend up to the masseter region. Following advancement of the flaps to the midline and direct approximation, the masseter muscle is exposed (Fig. 2.43).

JÄSCHE方法

这也是一种用于楔形，全下唇缺损再造的方法。肿瘤切除的切口呈V形由嘴角向下颏方向并向内凹陷。其将用于嘴-颏区域的自然再造并使再造的唇具有弹性。在两侧嘴角向外向下创建一条弧形切口并经过下颌边缘延伸到侧面颈部皮肤（图2.44）。通过向内侧旋转此尾部带蒂皮瓣可完成下唇的再造。

Method according to JÄSCHE

This method, too, is suited for reconstruction after excision of a wedge-shaped, total lower lip defect. The incision carried out to remove the tumor runs in a V-form from the oral commissure in a mental direction, in an inwardly concave form. The aim is to ensure a more natural reconstruction of the oral mental region, and, at the same time lend elasticity to the newly formed lip. Beginning from the oral commissure, two lateral, outwardly and downwardly arching incisions are made bilaterally. These incisions cross the jawline,

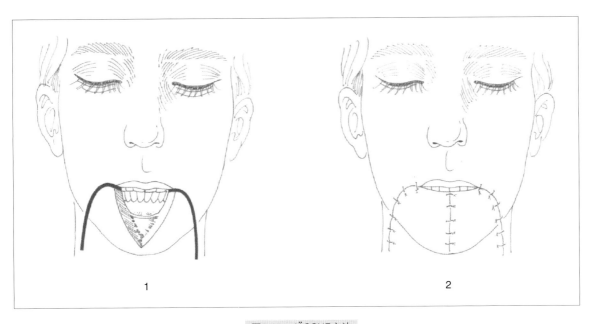

图2.44 JÄSCHE方法

Fig. 2.44 Method according to JÄSCHE

ending in the lateral neck skin (figs 2.44). Rotating these caudally pedicled flaps in a medial direction results in reconstruction of the lower lip.

根据HEURTAUX（1893）的改进，通过在V形切口底部切除的Burrow氏三角使得皮瓣的旋转变得简单。

According to HEURTAUX (1893), rotation can be carried out more easily by excising Burrow's triangles at the lower end of the V-shaped incision.

RIED方法

该方法也适合全下唇再造。从口角至下颌边缘设计两条向上凸起的弧形切口用于形成旋转皮瓣。在下颌缘高度水平作两侧松弛切口，使其向内几乎成直角状态（图2.45）。

Method according to RIED

This method is also indicated for a total loss of the lower lip. An arched, upwardly convex incision reaching from the commissure of the mouth up to the border of the lower jaw is made to create two rotational flaps. Level with the border of the lower jaw, two relaxing incisions run bilaterally in a medial (mental) direction almost at right angles (Fig. 2.45).

POLLOSSON方法（1893）

当通过V形切口切除全部下唇后，由口角向外侧水平作切口（A, B）并向下以一定角度延伸至下

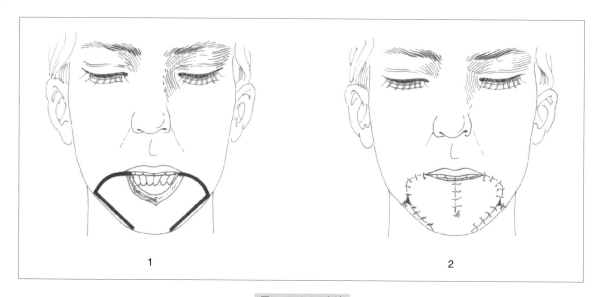

图2.45　RIED方法

Fig. 2.45　Method according to RIED

颌边缘（B, C）。AB和BC等长。通过向中间同时推进这两块面颊皮瓣将切口AB与BC顶部边缘缝合（图2.46）。为了再建唇红，将把AB段的下缘相对应的口腔黏膜向外旋转与皮肤缝合。

Method according to POLLOSSON (1893)

Following V-shaped excision of the full lower lip, a horizontal incision is developed from the oral commissure in a lateral direction (A, B) and continues in a downward angle to the jawline (B, C). The lines A, B and B, C have the same length. After shifting both buccal flaps towards the midline, the superior edges of A, B and B, C are sutured to each other on both sides (Fig. 2.46). For the lip vermilion, the oral mucosa corresponding to the inferior edge of A, B is rotated outwardly and sutured to the skin.

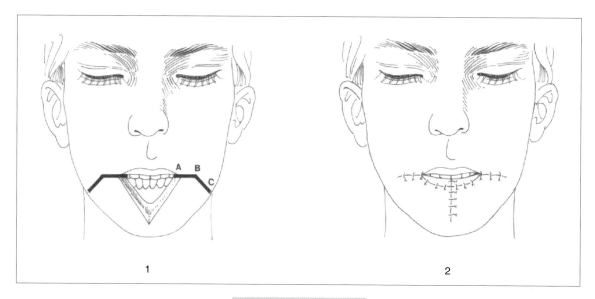

图2.46　POLLOSSON方法

Fig. 2.46　Method according to POLLOSSON

BERGER方法（1894）

BERGER方法与DIEFFENBACH（1845）近似，只是需两期完成。

Method according to BERGER (1894)

The BERGER technique is similar to that of DIEFFENBACH (1845), only that it is carried out in two stages.

第一期手术，将在嘴角向外侧创建一条大约3cm长的水平切口。此时面动脉将被结扎，口腔黏膜先不切断。在切开皮肤肌肉行黏膜下剥离后，将其在比外侧切口高1.5cm处切开。将黏膜瓣向外翻转，并再造唇红（图2.47-1）。

In the first operation, a horizontal incision is made from the oral commissure outwards to a length of about 3 cm. The facial artery is ligated and the oral mucosa is initially kept intact. After developing the myocutaneous incision the mucosa is freed submucously. The mucosa is then circumcised, also horizontally, but 1.5 cm higher than the external incision. This mucosal flap can then be flipped outwardly to reconstruct the lip vermilion (Fig. 2.47-1).

在手术期间将口裂的宽度扩大为原来的两倍。

This step of the operation lengthens the oral fissure by almost double.

在几周后，将进行第二次手术。将从新的口裂嘴角的终点向尾部创建一条3cm长、竖直的贯穿所

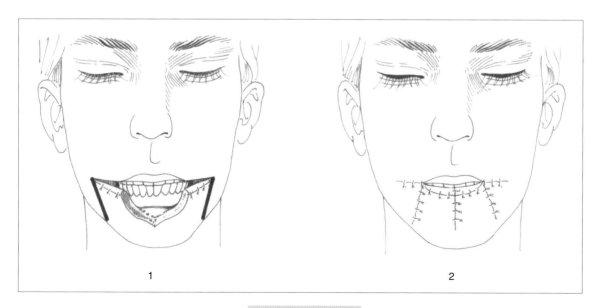

1　　　　　　　　　2

图2.47　BERGER方法

Fig. 2.47　Method according to BERGER

有颊部皮肤层的切口（图2.47-2）。所获取的皮瓣此时可向中部旋转用于重建下唇。之前还必须切除瘢痕。在颊部所生成的缺损可通过直接缝合来闭合。

In the second operation several weeks later, a 3cm long, vertical incision beginning from the end of the new commissure region is developed in a caudal direction through all thicknesses of the cheek (Fig. 2.47-2). The resulting flaps can now be rotated in a medial direction to reconstruct the lower lip. The scars must be excised beforehand. The secondary defects in the buccal region are closed by means of direct approximation.

ANGER方法（1877）

在完全切下下唇后，在切除创缘外下方作一向颏下直达颈区皮肤切口（C，D）并成直角返回下颌缘（D，E）。由此再造一个矩形皮瓣（B-C-D-E）（图2.48）。

Method according to ANGER (1877)

Following total resection of the lower lip, an auxiliary incision is made from the lateral caudal edge of the incision in a submental direction up to the skin of the neck (C-D) and back to the jawline at a right angle (D, E). This creates a rectangular flap (B-C-D-E) (Fig. 2.48).

伤口（B，C）将用于重建下唇（B-A），颏部和颈部软组织（C-D）将向C-A推进，E-D段向E-C段推进。

The edge of the wound (B-C) is used to reconstruct the lower lip (B-A), and the soft tissue of the chin

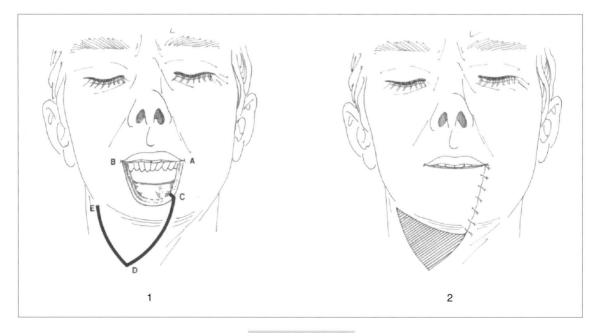

图2.48　ANGER方法

Fig. 2.48　Method according to ANGER

and neck (C-D) is shifted to C-A. The section E, D then becomes E-C.

这未处理的创面E-D-C可二期愈合（图2.48）。

The free wound area E-D-C is left to granulate secondarily (Fig. 2.48).

LEDRAN方法

在下唇局部矩形切除后，创口尾部稍稍内凹，再设计一平行于缺损皮肤的辅助切口。通过在剩余的皮瓣基部竖直的垂直切口，可以再建一块肌皮黏膜瓣，向上旋转此皮瓣可替代下唇（图2.49）。

Method according to LEDRAN

After box-shaped incision of a segment of the lower lip – the caudal wound edge is slightly concave– an auxiliary incision is made parallel to the skin defect. A perpendicular vertical incision on the remaining lip stump creates a rectangular myocutaneous-mucosal flap, which replaces the lower lip by means of upward rotation (Fig. 2.49).

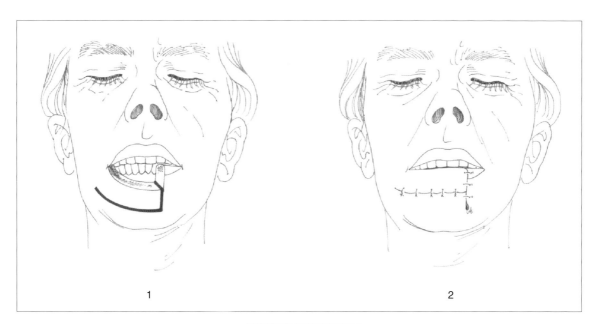

图2.49　LEDRAN方法

Fig. 2.49　Method according to LEDRAN

BERG方法

此方法与上篇所描述的LEDRAN方法近似。再建的辅助切口贯穿所剩余下唇–颏区域的所有层。首先向外倾斜，最后沿颏边缘逆行。同时通过颅侧旋转所再建的矩形皮瓣完成下唇的修复重建（图2.50）。

Method according to BERG

This method is similar to the previously described method according to LEDRAN. Here, though, the incision through all thicknesses of the remaining lower lip and mental region first runs outwardly on a diagonal, then retrograde along the jawline. Here, too, lower lip reconstruction is carried out via cranial rotation of the rectangular flap (Fig. 2.50).

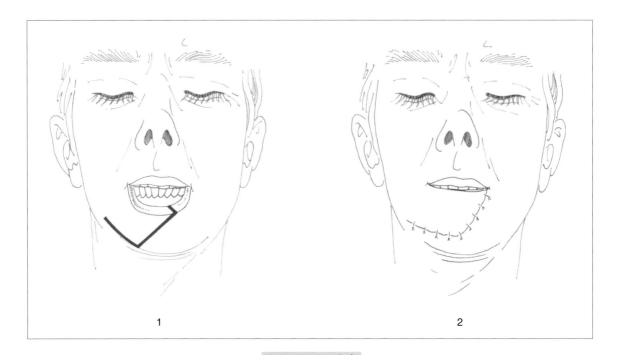

图2.50 BERG方法

Fig. 2.50 Method according to BERG

MONTET方法

在楔形切口切除下唇局部后，通过再造一个直角形，上部带蒂的黏膜肌皮瓣的上边宽度相当于楔形切除下唇缺损的宽度（图2.51）。

Method according to MONTET

Following wedge excision of a segment of the lower lip, a rectangular myocutaneous-mucosal flap is created; this flap remains cranially pedicled, and its cranial side corresponds to the wedge-shaped resection defect (Fig. 2.51).

DIEU-LAFOY方法和AUVERT方法

在楔形切口切除全部下唇后，首先作一从中间向下至颏部的垂直的切口。然后再作两条沿下颌边缘的水平切口，从而形成两个向上翻转的矩形皮瓣，产生颏下皮肤缺损可二期愈合（图2.52）。

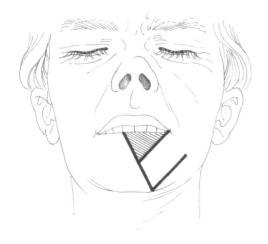

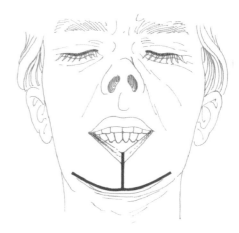

图2.51　MONTET方法

Fig. 2.51　Method according to MONTET

图2.52　DIEU-LAFOY方法

Fig. 2.52　Method according to DIEU-LAFOY

Method according to DIEU-LAFOY and AUVERT

After wedge excision of the entire lower lip, a vertical median incision is developed caudally. This incision ends at the mentum. Two additional horizontal incisions are made, which follow the jawline. This creates two rectangular flaps which are rotated upward. The resulting skin defect in the submental region is left to heal by secondary granulation (Fig. 2.52).

AUVERT方法与上述描述类似。所设计的辅助切口较长，中间的垂直切口直至甲状软骨。两侧辅助切口起于竖直切口末端上面2cm，向上逆行至下颌缘。两次产生的缺损可直接缝合（图2.53）。

The method according to AUVERT is similar to the one described above/to that of DIEU-LAFOY. The auxiliary incisions are longer; the median vertical incision ends at the thyroid cartilage and the lateral incisions begin at a point 2 cm. above the ending point of the vertical incision and run retrograde, ending at the jawline. This enables direct approximation of the secondary defect (Fig. 2.53).

VIGUERIE-MORGAN方法

在弧形切口切除下唇后，作一从口角向耳屏方向的切口。再在下颌骨下方作一平行于下颌的切口，从而形成一个可颅侧移动桥形皮瓣（图2.54）。

Method according to VIGUERIE-MORGAN

After curvilinear resection of the lower lip, an incision running towards the tragus is made through the oral commissure. A second parallel incision runs parallel to the lower jaw inferiorly to the base of the lower jaw. This creates a bridge flap which is advanced cranially to replace the lower lip (Fig. 2.54).

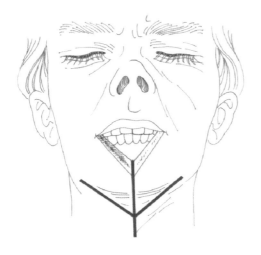

图2.53　AUVERT方法

Fig. 2.53　Method according to AUVERT

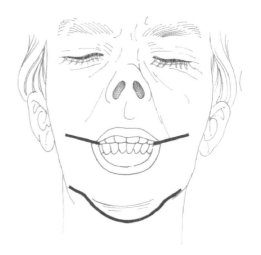

图2.54　VIGUERIE-MORGAN方法

Fig. 2.54　Method according to VIGUERIE-MORGAN

SZYMANOWSKI方法

SZYMANOWSKI对此方法进行了改进，在桥皮瓣的中央切除一块垂直椭圆形的肌皮区（图2.55）。

Method according to SZYMANOWSKI

SZYMANOWSKI modified this procedure by excising a vertical, oval-shaped myocutaneous area in the median of the bridge flap (Fig. 2.55).

SEDILLOT方法

此方法集合了SERRE，GUINARD，VIGUERIE，SEDILLOT和DIEFFENBACH的建议。

Method according to SEDILLOT

This method combines ideas from SERRE, GUINARD, VIGUERIE, SEDILLOT and DIEFFENBACH.

在完全切除下唇后作一条至下颌下的辅助切口和一条颅侧的平行于切除边缘的颊部切口（图2.56右侧）。通过移动黏膜肌皮瓣并向缺损处靠近来完成下唇再造。此方法的缺点在于不能修复下唇红，另外，口角修复也不令人满意。

Following resection of the entire lower lip, one auxiliary incision is made submentally, another is developed cranially, parallel to the margin of the buccal excision (Fig. 2.56, right side). Transposing the created myocutaneous-mucosal flap on both sides and suturing it into the defect reconstructs the lower lip. A drawback of this method is that it is not possible to reconstruct the lower lip vermilion. In addition, reconstruction of the oral commissure does not yield satisfactory results.

SEDILLOT方法的第二种方式

在盒式切除下唇后在缺损两侧形成两个至颏下的矩形头部带蒂皮瓣。这里的皮瓣只是两个皮肌皮瓣，其下部的黏膜将被保存。因为按照SEDILLOT方法进行的修复后，下唇黏膜将被保留（图2.57）。

Second method according to SEDILLOT (1848)

After box-shaped resection of the lower jaw, two right-angled, cranially-pedicled flaps which end submandibularly are made on both sides of the resection defect. These are purely myocutaneous flaps; the

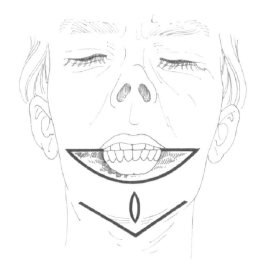

图2.55　SZYMNOWSKI方法

Fig. 2.55　Method according to SZYMNOWSKI

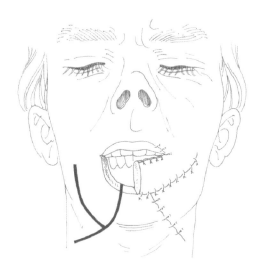

图2.56　SEDILLOT方法

Fig. 2.56　Method according to SEDILLOT

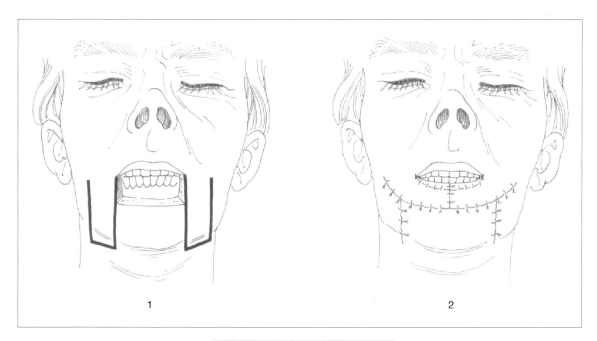

图2.57　SEDILLOT方法的第二种方式

Fig. 2.57　Second method of SEDILLOT

underlying mucosa is kept intact because this reconstructive method according to SEDILLOT preserves the mucosa (Fig. 2.57).

LALLEMANT方法（1824）

在下唇局部切除后作一条从嘴角区域开始的弧形切口B-A。再沿C-D作第二条辅助切口及沿D-E-A的第三条切口。在形成皮瓣E-F-H后，将其向颅侧翻转替代下唇（图2.58）。

Method according to LALLEMANT (1824)

After partial excision of the lower lip, a curvilinear incision is developed from the area of the commissure of the mouth along the line B-A. A second auxiliary incision is carried out from C to D, and a third incision along D-E-A. After creation of the flap E-F-H it is rotated cranially to replace the lower lip (Fig. 2.58).

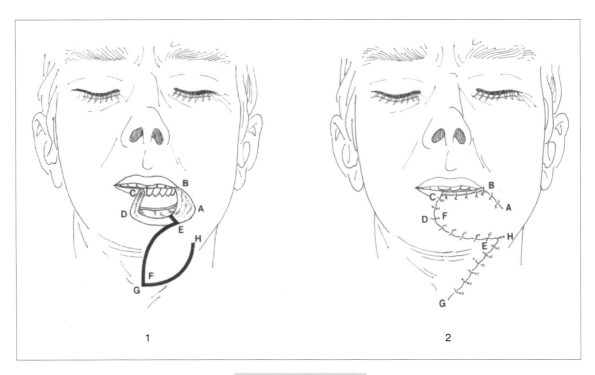

图2.58　LALLEMANT方法

Fig. 2.58　Method according to LALLEMANT

BLASIUS方法

图2.59：肿瘤通过V形切口切除。垂直于切口两边作两条延伸到下颌缘处再垂直转折至咬肌前缘的辅助切口（C-E和D-F）。由此形成的四角形皮瓣可颅侧旋转并间断缝合（C和D，E和F）。此外在颏区设计一条垂直的切口（H-K）。由此形成的皮瓣m和n用于覆盖旋转皮瓣所产生的二次创口。此方法是由RIGAUD（1841）和BLASIUS首次提出和描述的。

Method according to BLASIUS

Fig. 2.59: A V-shaped tumor excision is carried out. Two auxiliary incisions (C-E and D-F) are developed at a right angle to the first incision and, after having reached the jawline, they turn posteriorly at a right angle and continue up to the anterior edge of the masseter muscle. This produces two rectangular flaps which can be rotated cranially and adapted by means of interrupted sutures (C to D and E to F). An additional vertical incision is made in the mental area (H, K). The resulting flaps m and n serve to cover the secondary defect caused by flap rotation. The method was first described by RIGAUD (1841) and BLASIUS.

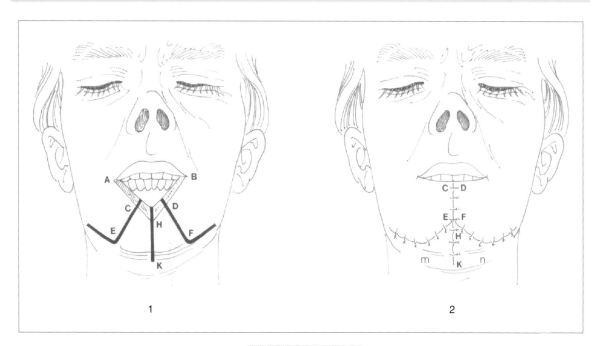

图2.59　BLASIUS方法

Fig. 2.59　Method according to BLASIUS

BUCHANAN-SYME方法

此方法中肿瘤也是由V形切口在下唇切除。切口的两条边（A，C和B，C）分别向尾部延伸形成一个X形切口。在两条切口的终点（D和F）各向两侧上方创建长约3cm的切口（D，E和F，G）。由此构建的皮瓣（A，C，D，E和B，C，F，G）向上翻转并将C，D段与C，F段相缝合。颏部所遗留的三角形D，C，F作为旋转皮瓣的支撑。

Method according to BUCHANAN-SYME

Here, too, tumor excision is carried out by means of a V-shaped resection of the lower lip. The sides of the V-shaped defect (A, C and B, C) are extended caudally direction to form an X-shaped incision. Two 3 cm.-long incisions are developed from the ending points of the X-shaped incision (D and F) in an upwardly lateral direction (D, E and F, G). The resulting flaps (A, C, D, E and B, C, F, G) are then rotated upward and the lines C, D and C, F sutured to-gether. The remaining mental triangle D, C, F serves as support for the rotated flaps.

三角形C，G，F和C，D，E可二期愈合（图2.60）。

The remaining triangles C, G, F and C, D, E are left to heal by secondary granulation (Fig. 2.60).

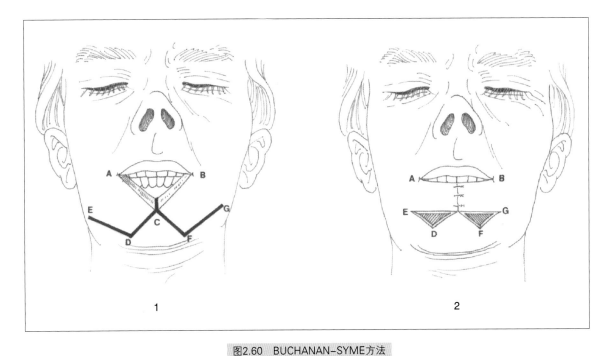

图2.60　BUCHANAN-SYME方法

Fig. 2.60　Method according to BUCHANAN-SYME

TRELAT方法（1861）

肿瘤的切除是通过口裂延长线方向上的两条35mm长的切口（A，B），最后斜向下的42mm长的第二条切口和平行于原下唇唇红的30mm长的切口（C到c）。通过作一条垂直向下并最终延伸至下颌缘的辅助切口（C-D），C-D长30mm并超出颏边缘。再作一条长28mm的水平松弛切口（D-E和d-e）。由此形成矩形皮瓣。其向上推进并相互缝合（C点和c点，D点和d点）。供皮区可二期愈合（图2.61）。

Method according to TRELAT (1861)

The tumor is removed by means of two 35 mm.-long incisions developed in the axis of the oral commissure (A, B). A second, 42 mm.-long incision follows, running in an oblique, downward direction, as well as a 30 mm.-long incision running parallel to what used to be the vermilion of the lip (C to c). 30 mm.-long, vertical auxiliary incisions run downward, along the jawline (C-D) and C-D, and then traverse the jawline; 28 mm.-long, horizontal relaxing incisions (D-E and d-e) are made. This forms two rectangular flaps which can be transposed upward and sutured together (the point C is sutured to c, and D to d). The donor site heals by secondary granulation (Fig. 2.61).

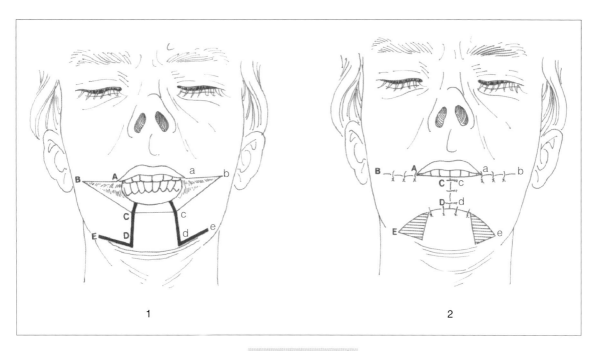

图2.61　TRELAT方法

Fig. 2.61　Method according to TRELAT

LANGENBECK方法

肿瘤所在下唇通过一条向上凹面的弧形切口（A，C，B）除去。之后切开一个位于颏部并可向上旋转的皮瓣（C，E，F，D）。颏肌区域保留下来的皮肌区（E，C，A）作为支撑用于抵抗由于瘢痕原因造成的再造下唇的尾部偏移（图2.62）。

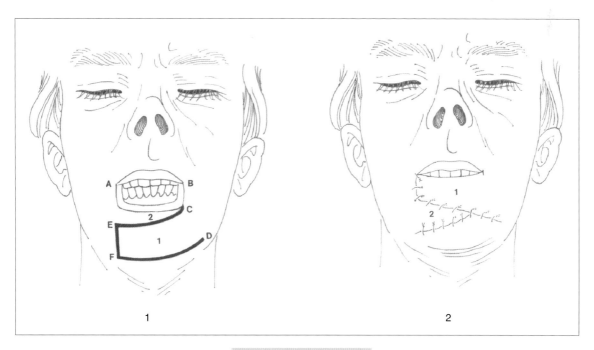

图2.62　LANGENBECK方法

Fig. 2.62　Method according to LANGENBECK

Method according to LANGENBECK

The malignant lower lip segment is removed by means of an upwardly concave, curvilinear incision (A, C, B). Then a flap is circumcised (C, E, F, D), which is elevated in the mental region and rotated upward. The remaining myocutaneous area (E, C, A) in the region of the mentalis muscle serves as support against caudal shifting of the reconstructed lip caused by scar tissue (figs. 2.62).

LAORDEN方法（1873）

下唇的肿瘤通过V形切口切除。切口单侧向尾部至下颌边缘延伸。在此切口末端向中间作第二切口与其成锐角并与A—B段平行。最终将所形成的三角形皮瓣向上旋转。供皮区同样可二期愈合（图2.63）。

Method according to LAORDEN (1873)

The lower lip tumor is removed by means of a V-shaped incision; one side of the V is lengthened caudally up to the jawline. At the end of this incision, a second acute-angled incision runs medially parallel to the line A-B. Then, the thus created triangular flap is rotated upward. The donor area is also left to heal by secondary granulation (Fig. 2.63).

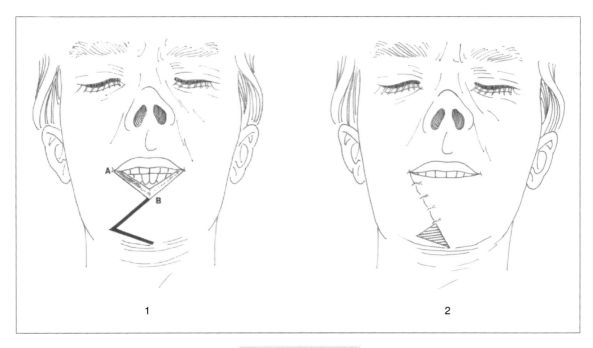

图2.63 LAORDEN方法

Fig. 2.63 Method according to LAORDEN

LANDREAU方法

盒式切口切除肿瘤后，在下唇缺损所在处颊侧通过两个同心圆弧形切口构建一个旋转皮瓣，并将其向上方中间旋转（图2.64-1）。

Method according to LANDREAU

Following box-shaped resection of the lower lip, two concentric, curvilinear incisions are made laterally to the lower jaw defect in the buccal area to form a rotational flap which is rotated upward in a medial direction (Fig. 2.64-1).

图2.64-2显示了最终的效果，供皮区缺损可通过直接缝合来修复。

Fig. 2.64-2 shows the end result and coverage of the defect in the donor area by means of direct approximation.

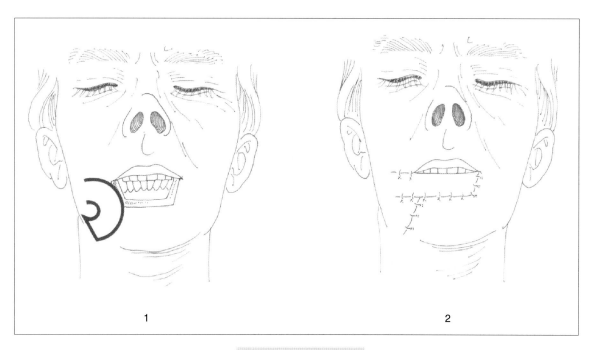

图2.64 LANDREAU方法

Fig. 2.64 Method according to LANDREAU

OLLIER方法

肿瘤及其所在的下唇通过盒式切口切除。A，B，C，D表示了缺损范围的边界。然后作一条弧形切口（C，D，E）。再作第二条切口L，M，N与第一条切口（C,D,E）平行。两条切口的间距与下唇缺损的高度相吻合。由此将形成的桥形皮瓣向颅侧旋转，同时C，E，D皮区将可预防再造的下唇向下移位。形成的二次损伤可通过二次愈合（图2.65）。

Method according to OLLIER

The tumor or the lower lip is removed by means of a box-shaped resection. The points A, C, D and B outline the edges of the defect. There follows a curvilinear incision (C, E, D). A further incision L, M, N runs parallel to the initial curved line (C, E, D). The distance between C, D and L, M, N corresponds to the height of the lower lip defect. The resulting bridge flap is rotated in a cranial direction; the area C, E, D serves to prevent postoperative caudal shifting of the newly formed lip. The resulting secondary defect heals by second intention (Fig. 2.65).

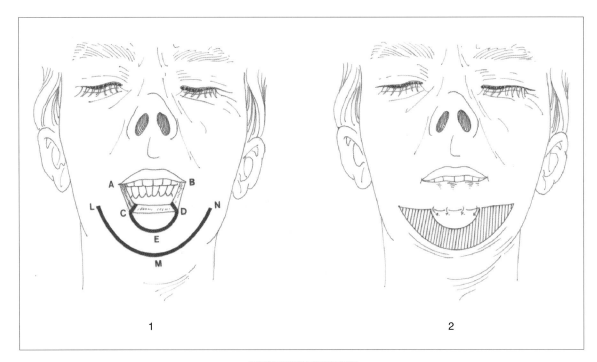

图2.65　OLLIER方法

Fig. 2.65　Method according to OLLIER

LARGER方法（1894）
根据此方法可运用鼻唇沟区域的颊–上唇皮瓣来再造下唇。

Method according to LARGER (1894)
In this technique, reconstruction of the lower lip is performed using a compound buccal and upper lip flap from the region of the nasolabial groove.

从上唇外侧1/3处向上方外侧作一条切口A，B，此时上唇须完全切开。从此切口末端再作一条向下方的切口（B，C）。上唇红（A，D）最终切除，皮瓣（A，B，C，D）移动并向下旋转。将推进的口腔黏膜在推进皮瓣的上缘缝合来再造下唇红。供区可直接缝合（图2.66）。

The incision A, B is made beginning from a lateral one third of the upper lip and developed in an upwardly lateral direction. The lower lip is cut through all thicknesses. A second incision (B, C) runs from the end of the first in a laterally caudal direction. The lip vermilion (A, D) is then excised; the flap (A, B, C, D) is mobilized and rotated downward. The mobilized oral mucosa is sutured to the superior edge of the transposition flap (B, C) to reconstruct the lip vermilion. The donor region is closed via direct suture approximation (Fig. 2.66).

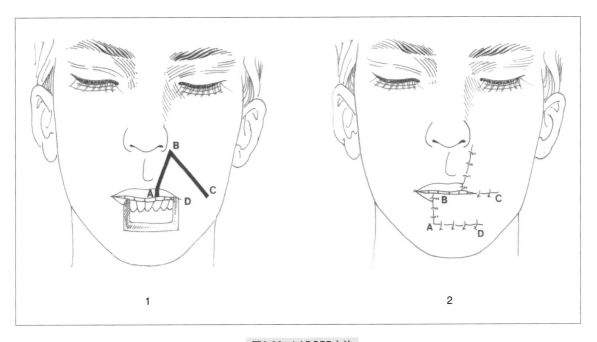

图2.66　LARGER方法

Fig. 2.66　Method according to LARGER

DELPECH方法（1823）

这是一种用颈部皮肤来再造下唇的方法。

Method according to DELPECH (1823)

This technique uses the skin of the neck to reconstruct the lower lip.

再造术可通过180°旋转皮瓣来实现。此方法经常导致皮瓣坏死。另外，此下唇再造法还显示出强烈的收缩趋势和尾部偏移以及相应的唾液失禁。出于对该法历史价值的尊重在这里对此略作描述。

Reconstruction is carried out via 180° rotation of the flap. This method often leads to flap necrosis. Furthermore, a lower lip reconstructed according to this technique displays a significant shrinkage and caudal sagging together with corresponding salivary incontinence. This method is described here out of purely historical interest.

在切除肿瘤及全部下唇后（图2.67-1），以弧形切口形成一个从颏下到胸骨的颈皮瓣，其基底在颏下。游离皮瓣后，将下部1/3处沿AB线向内反折并与重叠的皮肤缝合。此两层皮瓣绕基部旋转180°。形成的下唇由三层组成，内外部都由皮肤覆盖。在第一次手术恢复若干星期后，基部将被切断（图2.67-2）。

After removing the tumor or the entire lower lip (Fig. 2.67-1) a neck skin flap is formed by means of a curvilinear incision from the submental region up to the manubrium of the sternum. Its basis is submental. After freeing the flap, its inferior third is swiveled inwards along the axis A, B and adapted to the overlying skin. After mobilization, this two-layered flap is now rotated around its base by 180°. The reconstructed lower lip now consists of three layers and covered with skin inside and out. After ingrowth of the flap, the base is divided severed several weeks after the first operation (Fig. 2.67-2).

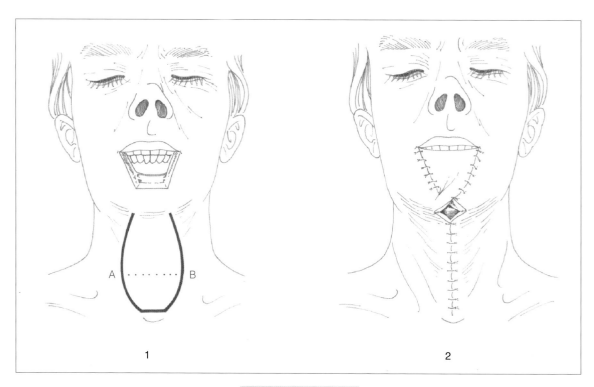

图2.67　DELPECH方法

Fig. 2.67　Method according to DELPECH

VOISIN方法（1835）

此方法与DELPECH方法的区别在于颈部皮瓣的外形为梯形。皮瓣底部宽于基部，长约6cm，下部切口水平位于甲状软骨。然后皮瓣绕基部旋转180°。

Method according to VOISIN (1835)

This method differs from that of DELPECH consists in the development of the neck skin flap in a trapezoid form. The inferior edge of the flap is wider than its base and approximately 6 cm. long. The inferior incision is carried out horizontally level with the thyroid cartilage, then the flap is turned in its base by 180°.

下唇内侧将不重建，并让其二期愈合。这就造成比DELPECH更严重的瘢痕引起的再造下唇的收

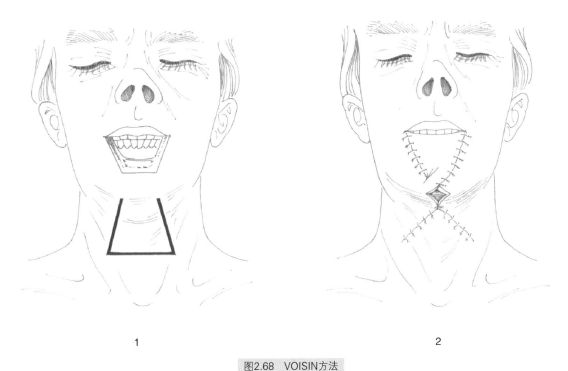

1
2

图2.68　VOISIN方法

Fig. 2.68　Method according to VOISIN

缩（图2.68）。

Reconstruction of the interior of the lower lip does not take place. The defect heals by secondary granulation. This causes a yet stronger pull of the scar in the reconstructed lower lip than in the DELPECH technique (Fig. 2.68).

ANDREWS方法（1964）

此方法适用于下唇缺损为1/3～2/3唇宽度的病例。

Method according to ANDREWS (1964)

This method is indicated when the lower lip defect involves between one and two thirds of the width of the lower lip.

图2.69-1描绘了下唇肿瘤通过贯穿所有皮肤层的楔形切口切除。在楔形切口两侧分别作切口X，Y，Z和矩形皮瓣A，B，C，D和B，E，O，C。此时AB段、BC段、CD段、XZ段以及YZ段等长。

Fig. 2.69-1 illustrates lip tumor removal by means of a wedge-shaped incision through all thicknesses of the lip. In the region of the lateral, wedge-shaped incision the line of incision for X, Y, Z and for the rectangular flaps A, B, C, D and B, E, O, C are shown. The length of A, B equals B, C, equals C, D, equals X, Z and Y, Z.

在楔形切口边缘切除四边形BEOC。皮瓣A，B，C，D此时向上旋转，皮瓣Z，Y，O向下牵引。

Next to the wedge-shaped region, the rectangle B, E, O, C is removed. The flap A, B, C, D is then rotated upward and the flap Z, Y, O is brought down.

如图2.69-1所示Y与D，X，B相缝合。唇红由口腔前庭黏膜重建。

In accordance with Fig. 2.69-1, Y is sutured to D and X to B. The vermilion is reconstructed using the mucosa of the oral vestibule.

图2.69-2显示了最终的效果。

Fig. 2.69-2 shows the end result.

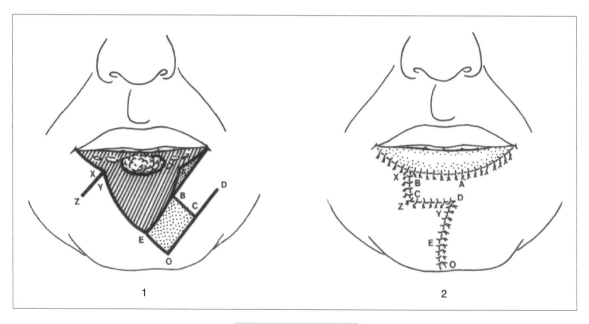

图2.69　ANDREWS方法

Fig. 2.69　Method according to ANDREWS

OWENS方法（1944）

此方法用于修复全下唇缺损。图2.70-1描绘了肿瘤切除后的状态以及在两侧作由表层表情肌和皮肤组成的颊皮瓣的切口。血管供应是下唇动脉通过唇蒂来完成的。虚线显示口腔黏膜的切口。

Method according to OWENS (1944)

This method is described for replacement of the entire lip. Fig. 2.70-1 shows the appearance after removal of the tumor. It also shows the line of incision which creates two lateral buccal flaps consisting of skin and superficial mimetic muscle. Vascular supply on each side occurs via one of the labial pedicles of the inferior labial artery. The dotted line shows the planned intraoral incision of the mucosa.

图2.70-2显示了颊黏膜瓣的设计。通过向中间旋转两侧此颊黏膜瓣能够完成唇红的重建。两个垂直的颊肌瓣向中间颅侧旋转至下唇缺损处。

Fig. 2.70-2 shows the development of a mucosal flap from the buccal mucosa. After rotation of these

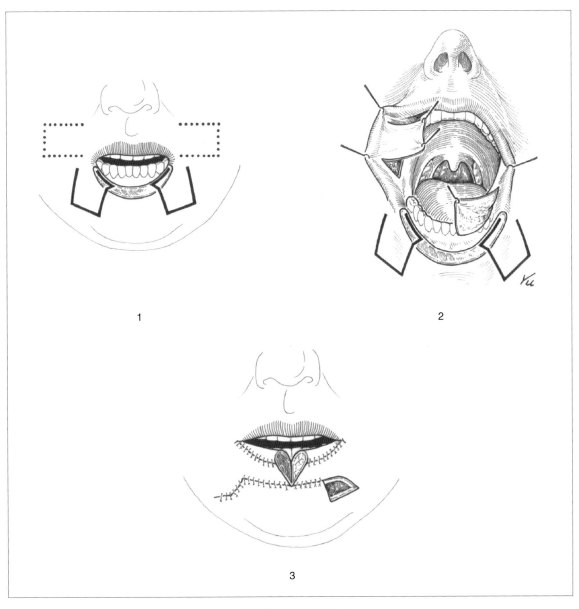

1

2

3

图2.70　OWENS方法

Fig. 2.70　Method according to OWENS

bilateral buccal mucosa flaps medially, they can be used to reconstruct the lip vermilion. Each of the vertical buccal myocutaneous flaps are rotated medially in a cranial direction and brought into the lower lip defect.

图2.70-3描绘了下唇再造后的状态和右边供区缺损缝合状况。

Fig. 2.70-3 shows the appearance after reconstruction of the lip vermilion and closure of the donor area defect on the right side.

外侧旋转皮瓣
此技术适用于全部下唇缺损的修复。

Lateral Rotation Flaps
This technique is also suitable defect coverage after total loss of the lower lip.

图2.71-1表述了下唇切除范围和两个旋转皮瓣的切口线。基于下唇动脉的带蒂皮瓣b旋转180° 到达缺损处并与旋转90° 的皮瓣b'缝合。此皮瓣由皮肤和肌肉组织组成并通过唇动脉分支供血。

The excision area of the lower lip and the line of incision to create two rotation flaps are shown in Fig. 2.71-1. The pedicled flap b, which is based on the inferior labial artery is rotated into the defect by 180° and sutured to the flapb′, which has previously been rotated by 90°. This flap contains skin and muscle tissue and is supplied by branches of the labial artery.

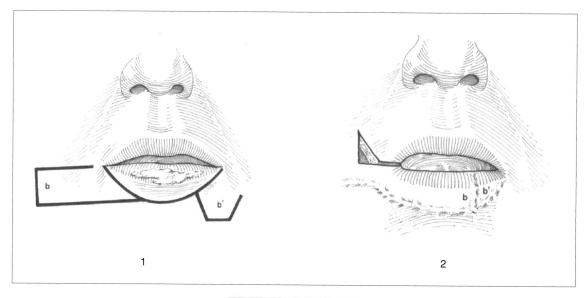

图2.71　外侧旋转皮瓣方法

Fig. 2.71　Lateral Rotation Flap Technique

此方法的缺点在于右侧产生的多余组织需要通过二次手术切除（图2.71-2）。

The drawback of this method is that surplus tissue on the right side must be reduced in a second operation (Fig. 2.71-2).

"Bi-lobed flap" 方法
此方法可追溯到1953年由ZIMANY首次提出。

The Bi-lobed Flap Technique
This method dates back to ZIMANY who first described it in 1953.

它适用于下唇的完全再造。

The method is indicated for total reconstruction of the lower lip.

图2.72-1描述了下唇切除的切口和在面颊形成一个双叶形的旋转皮瓣。垂直方向的皮瓣面积大于与其90°相交的水平方向的皮瓣。

Fig. 2.72-1 shows the incision line incised for excision of the entire lower lip and development of a bilobed rotation flap from the buccal region. The vertically directed flap A is larger than the diagonally horizontal second flap situated at a 90° angle from the first flap.

在切除下唇后旋转由皮肤组织和皮下组织组成的皮瓣A至缺损处（图2.72-2），供区缺损由皮瓣B覆盖，所产生的二次缺损可通过直接缝合关闭。

After excision of the lower lip (Fig. 2.72-2), the flap A which consists of skin and subcutaneous tissue is rotated into the lower lip defect. The donor area is covered with flap B. The resulting residual defect can be closed by direct approximation.

图2.72-3显示了初步的术后状态。愈合期后需进行二次手术以切断皮瓣A的蒂部。

Fig. 2.72-3 shows the interim end result. After a period of ingrowth, a second operation is necessary, in which the pedicle of flap A is divided.

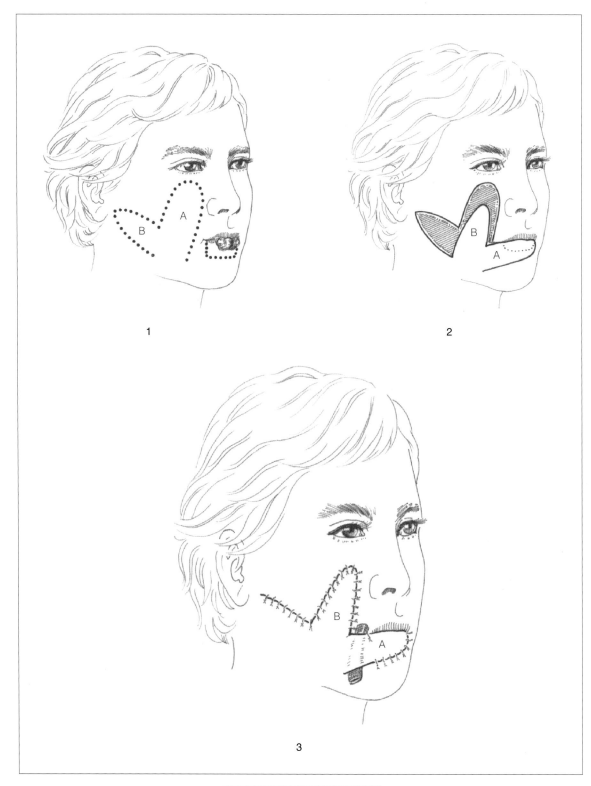

图2.72 "Bi-lobed-flap" 方法

Fig. 2.72 Method according to "Bi-lobed-flap"

BRUNS鼻唇皮瓣整形术

1859年由BRUNS提出了运用鼻唇皮瓣来再造下唇单侧缺损的方法。

Nasolabial flap plastic surgery according to BRUNS

The use of a nasolabial flap for reconstruction of the lateral segment of the lower lip was described in 1859 by BRUNS.

图2.73-1描述了下唇切除后由相邻鼻唇沟区域形成一个下部带蒂的旋转皮瓣的切口。通过90°旋转鼻唇沟皮瓣使其覆盖下唇缺损处。唇红通过颊黏膜重建。鼻唇沟区域所产生的二次损伤可直接缝合。图2.73-2显示了治疗的最终状态。

Fig. 2.73-1 outlines the part of the lower lip which will be excised and the incision line for the development of a rotation flap from the adjacent nasolabial region with a caudal pedicle. The nasolabial flap can then be rotated by 90° into the defect. Lower red lip reconstruction is performed using the buccal mucosa. The secondary defect in the nasolabial area can be closed by direct approximation. Fig. 2.73-2 shows the final result.

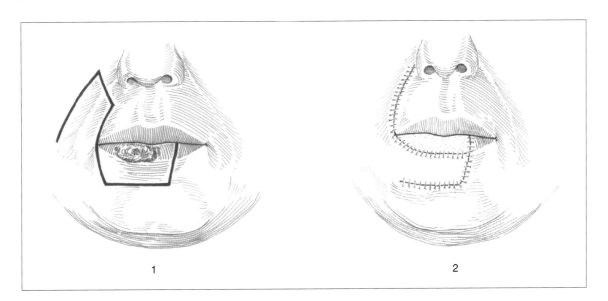

图2.73　BRUNS方法

Fig. 2.73　Method according to BRUNS

改良的鼻唇皮瓣

此方法适用于下唇全部缺损的病症。图2.74-1描绘了下唇区域的完全缺损以及在鼻唇区域一侧设计的切口并向另一侧延伸至面颊。切口贯穿所有面颊层。通过旋转这两块皮瓣可完成重建下唇。图2.74-2描绘了此方法的最终状态。

Modified Nasolabial Flap

This is indicated for total loss of the lower lip. Fig. 2.74-1 shows the total defect in the lower lip region and the line of incision which is situated in the nasolabial region on one side and which runs laterally into the cheek on the opposite side. The incision is made through all thicknesses of the cheek. Reconstruction of the lower lip is carried out by rotating both of these flaps into the defect area. Fig. 2.74-2 shows the final result.

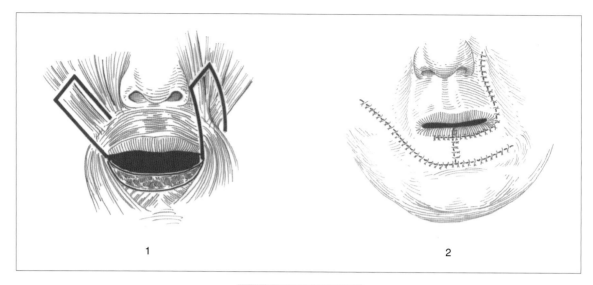

图2.74　改良的鼻唇皮瓣

Fig. 2.74　Modified Nasolabial Flap

BRUNS方法双侧鼻唇皮瓣

此手术技术同样适用于下唇完全缺损的再造。

Bilateral nasolabial flap according to BRUNS

This operative technique is also indicated to fully reconstruct the lower lip.

图2.75-1描绘了切除有恶性病变的下唇的切口线以及形成两个下部带蒂的全层鼻唇瓣切口线。每个瓣都以90°向中间旋转至缺损处。

Fig. 2.75-1 shows the line of incision to excise the lower lip carrying a malignant change, and the development of two nasolabial flaps with a caudal pedicle through all thicknesses. Each flap can be rotated by 90° median and inset into the defect.

图2.75-2描绘了手术的最终状态。唇红可通过颊部黏膜重建。

Fig. 2.75-2 shows the final result. The lip vermilion has been reconstructed from the buccal mucosa.

这种方法的最大缺点在于因供区直接缝合导致的上唇张力大。另外，两侧口轮匝肌肌肉组织与运动神经的联系会被切断。这将破坏嘴的关闭功能。同时此方法还会造成大面积的瘢痕区。

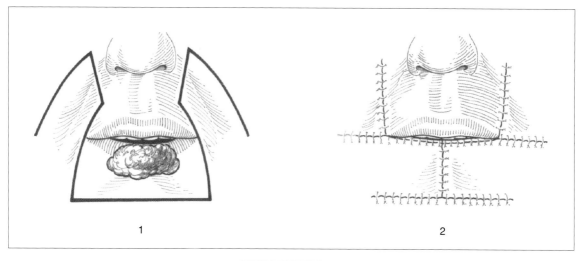

图2.75　BRUNS方法

Fig. 2.75　Method according to BRUNS

One disadvantage of this method is the upper lip tension ensuing from direct approximation of the donor defects. Furthermore, the muscle of the orbicularis oris is severed bilaterally, together with the motor nerves. This restricts the function of the oral sphincter This method also causes extensive scar formation.

SZYMANOWSKI方法

此方法适用于下唇完全缺损以及同时伴随邻近唇黏膜至龈唇沟缺损。图2.76-1描绘了下唇全厚度矩形切除的切口线以及在鼻唇沟外侧形成皮瓣的切口。

Method according to SZYMANOWSKI

This method is indicated for complete loss of the lower lip and simultaneous loss of the adjacent labial mucosa extending to the gingivolabial sulcus. Fig. 2.76-1 shows the development of the rectangular line of incision to resect the lower lip through all thicknesses, and the creation of the flap laterally from the nasolabial groove on both sides.

在右侧可部分保留嘴角以及相邻唇红。面颊区的皮瓣近似为矩形。皮瓣的宽度与缺损高度相等。脸颊黏膜两侧切开略宽于皮肌部分。这一超出的黏膜部分将用于重建新的下唇红。

On the right side, part of the oral commissure and the adjacent lower lip vermilion can be preserved. The flaps from the buccal region are nearly rectangular. Flap width corresponds to the height of the defect. The incision of the buccal mucosa is laterally larger than that of the cutaneous muscle. These extensions of the mucosa serve to reconstruct the lost lip vermilion.

图2.76-2描绘了两侧皮瓣设计状态，图2.76-3显示了最终状态。

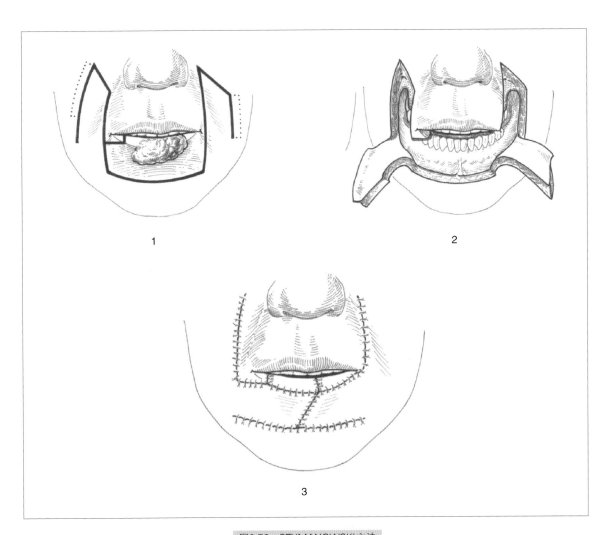

1   2

3

图2.76 SZYMANOWSKI方法

Fig. 2.76 Method according to SZYMANOWSKI

Fig. 2.76-2 shows the appearance after development of the bilateral flaps, Fig. 2.76-3 shows the final result.

此方法的优点在于一次性在完成下唇再造的同时完成唇红的修复。然而此方法同时也会在两侧下唇和鼻唇区域造成大的瘢痕区。表情肌在获取皮瓣时会受到损伤，进而影响到唇的功能。90°旋转皮瓣后造成的"猫耳"必须通过二次手术来矫正。

The advantage of this technique is that it permits defect coverage of the entire lower lip and simultaneous reconstruction of the lip vermilion. In addition it is one-stage. However, this reconstructive method leaves extensive scarring on both sides of the lower lip and nasolabial area. Excision of the flaps restricts the action of the mimetic muscles and causes lip dysfunction. The "pig-ear or dog-ear" resulting from flap rotation by 90° may require secondary correction.

FUJIMORI岛状皮瓣方法（1980）

此方法适用于下唇全层整复。

Gate Flap Method according to FUJIMORI (1980)

This method is also suited for total reconstruction of the lower lip through all thicknesses.

图2.77-1描绘了切除大的下唇肿瘤的切口线。矩形切口通过两侧嘴角（Bb-Dd）。切口边缘尾部可能延伸至颏唇沟。两侧水平边缘BO距离5～10mm，BD段长度约为3cm。

Fig. 2.77-1 demonstrates the incision for removal of the extensive lower lip tumor. The rectangular excision runs through the oral commissure bilaterally (Bb-Dd). The caudal edge of the excision is situated, if possible, in the mentolabial sulcus. The lateral horizontal edge of the resection BO is usually situated 5~10 mm. The incision BD is approximately 3cm long.

然后沿AB和AC切开并贯穿皮肤和肌肉。黏膜切口沿虚线AB，AMC。打点区域将做皮下剥离。

Then, incisions are developed through the skin and muscle layers along the lines AB and AC. The mucosa is placed along the interrupted lines AB, AMC. The dotted areas are undermined subcutaneously.

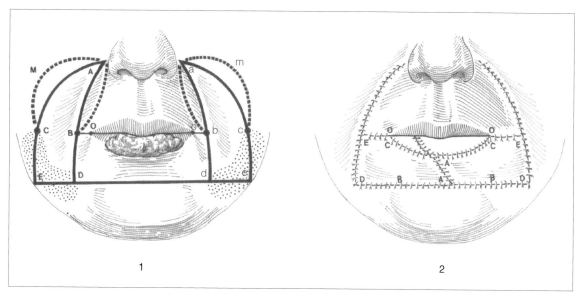

图2.77 FUJIMORI方法

Fig. 2.77 Method according to FUJIMORI

图2.77-2描绘了手术的最终效果。

Fig. 2.77-2 shows the final result.

KARAPANDZIC含动脉血管推进皮瓣方法

此方法适用于下唇次全切除再造的病例。图2.78-1描绘了使用盒形切口切除下唇肿瘤以及用于形成两个旋转皮瓣的弧形切口。

Arterialized local flap according to KARAPANDZIC

This method is indicated for subtotal lower lip reconstruction. Fig. 2.78-1 shows the box-shaped incision to excise a lower lip tumor and the curvilinear incision for the creation of two rotation flaps.

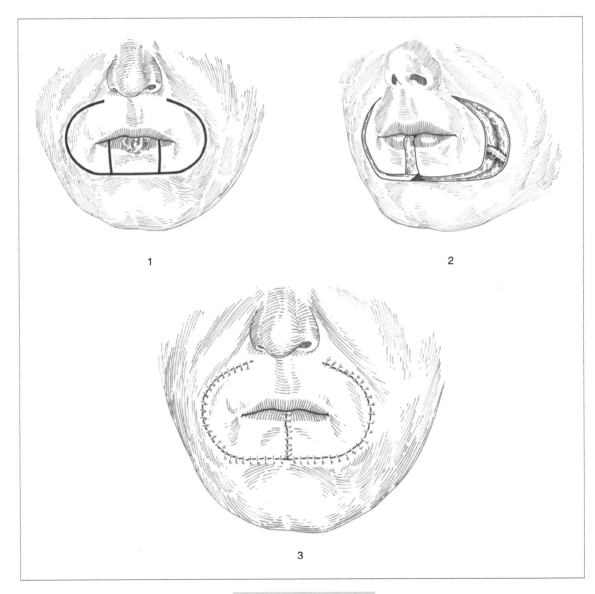

图2.78　KARAPANDZIC方法

Fig. 2.78　Method according to KARAPANDZIC

图2.78-2描绘了下唇肿瘤切除并形成下唇-面颊-旋转皮瓣后的状态。切开贯穿皮肤和肌肉组织，保持黏膜不受破坏。面部血管仔细地保护起来。通过转移这两个皮瓣并直接缝合后可完成下唇组织的重建。唇红可通过旋转邻近黏膜来重建。图2.78-3描绘了手术的最终状态。

Fig. 2.78-2 shows the appearance after tumor excision and incision of the lower lip-buccal rotation flaps. The incision traverses the skin and muscle; the mucosa remains intact. The facial blood vessels are meticulously preserved. After mobilization of both of these flaps, the lower lip substance is reconstructed by direct approximation. The red lip is reconstructed from the adjacent mucosa by rotation. Fig. 2.78-3 shows the final result.

KARAPANDZIC方法（1974）
该方法也可用于下唇全层缺损的重建。

Method according to KARAPANDZIC (1974)
This is another method which is indicated for reconstruction of a lower lip defect through all thicknesses.

图2.79-1描绘了整个下唇通过盒形切口切除以及形成向下向唇沟外侧，旋转皮瓣的切口。在切取皮瓣时，两边都必须保留面部动脉。皮瓣形成后，可向中间旋转来重建下唇。下唇红可采用两颊黏膜修复。

Fig. 2.79-1 outlines the box-shaped incision for removal of the total lower lip as well and the incision for creating lateral rotation flaps caudally to the nasolabial area. When incising the flap, care must be taken to

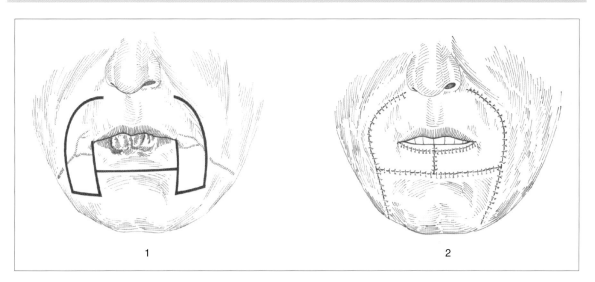

1   2

图2.79　KARPANDZIC方法

Fig. 2.79　Method according to KARPANDZIC

preserve the facial artery bilaterally. The flap is raised and then rotated medially to reconstruct the lower lip. The lip vermilion is formed from the buccal mucosa.

图2.79-2显示了最后的状态。

Fig. 2.79-2 shows the final result.

STEIN方法（1848）
该方法采用人中的两块全层三角皮瓣来重建楔形下唇缺损。采用该方法的指标为病变长达至下唇宽度的50%。

Method according to STEIN (1848)
This technique reconstructs a wedge-shaped lower lip defect by means of two triangular flaps through all layers, which are created from the philtrum of the upper lip. The technique is indicated when up to 50% of the breadth of the lower lip is involved.

图2.80-1描绘了由上唇人中形成两个全层三角皮瓣的切口。

Fig. 2.80-1 shows the incision lines to form 2 triangular flaps through all thicknesses of the upper lip philtrum.

唇红中的唇动脉的分支来营养皮瓣。

These flaps are nourished by branches of the labial artery in the lip vermilion.

图2.80-2描绘了皮瓣通过旋转置入下唇缺损处并且缝合。

In Fig. 2.80-2 the small flaps have been inset into the lower lip defect by rotation and sutured.

在第一次手术2～4周后的第二次介入治疗中，皮瓣蒂部将被切断并修复唇红。该方法的缺点无疑是会破坏人中的结构。

In a second operation taking place from two to four weeks after the first one, the pedicle of the flap is divided and the red lip reconstructed. No doubt the destruction of the philtrum's structure represents a disadvantage of this method.

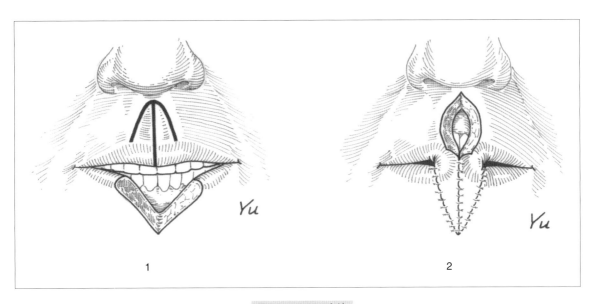

图2.80　STEIN方法

Fig. 2.80　Method according to STEIN

根据KAZANJIAN和ROOPENIAN对于STEIN手术的修改（1954）

　　此方法也可用于下唇缺损在50%上的情况。与STEIN手术不同，将从人中两侧形成皮瓣，从而保留人中结构（图2.81-1）。

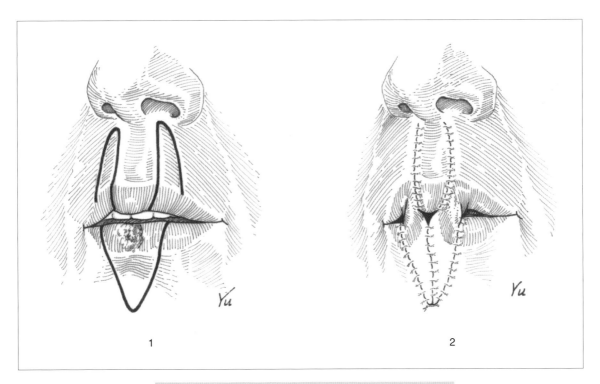

图2.81　根据KAZANJIAN和ROOPENIAN对于STEIN手术的修改

Fig. 2.81　Modification of the STEIN Operation according to KAZANJIAN and ROOPENIAN

Modification of the STEIN operative technique according to KAZANJIAN and ROOPENI-AN (1954)

Here, too, coverage of a lower lip defect of 50% is possible. In contradistinction to the STEIN operation, the bilateral flaps are taken laterally from the philtrum on both sides in order to maintain its structure (Fig. 2.81-1).

图2.81-2描绘了两个皮瓣向下旋转并覆盖所要修补的缺损处。同样该方法也需要在2～4周后进行二次手术。

In Fig. 2.81-2 both flaps have been rotated down and inset into the defect. Here, too, a second operation is performed two to four weeks later.

ASHLEY方法（1955）

下唇缺损达到下唇宽度一半的情况下，可采用该方法。图2.82-1描绘了用于切除下唇肿瘤的弧形切口。

Method according to ASHLEY (1955)

This method is indicated for lower lip defects which involve up to one half of the lip's breadth. Fig. 2.82-1 shows the curvilinear incision line for lower lip tumor excision.

位于上唇部分的切口在保护嘴角的前提下首先穿过上唇红，沿唇红/唇白边界一小段后，向上部外侧延伸至鼻唇沟，并沿此纹向下。当此皮瓣形成后，将其旋转90°至下唇缺损部位（图2.82-2）。

The incision line in the upper lip segment runs initially through the vermilion of the upper lip, but preserves the mouth angle; it then briefly follows the border between lip red and lip white and then rises laterally until it reaches the nasolabial groove; it then follows the nasolabial groove in a caudal direction. The developed flap is then rotated at an angle of 90° angle into the lower lip defect (Fig. 2.82-2).

在之后的二次手术中，将皮瓣蒂部切开，所剩的皮瓣部分向上部外侧旋转，从而再造出完整的上唇红。下唇红则由口腔前庭的黏膜形成（图2.82-3）。

In a second operation, the flap pedicle is separated; the circumcised part of the flap is rotated laterally upward and used to fully reconstruct the vermilion of the upper lip. The vermilion of the lower lip is reconstructed using mucosa of the inferior vestibule (Fig. 2.82-3).

图2.82-4描绘了最终状态。

Fig. 2.82-4 shows the final result.

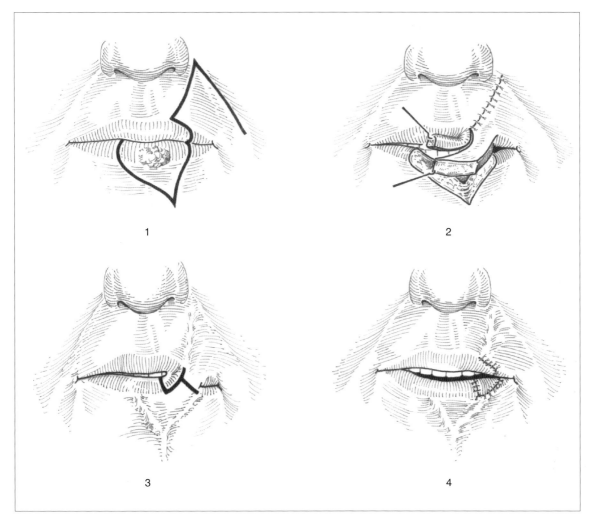

图2.82　ASHLEY方法

Fig. 2.82　Method according to ASHLEY

ABBE皮瓣

根据ABBE（1898）方法，将采用上唇部分的皮瓣来再造下唇。此皮瓣由带有唇动脉的唇红区的细长基部来供血。

ABBE Flaps

In the method according to ABBE (1898) a part of the upper lip is used to reconstruct the lower lip. This upper lip segment is nourished via the narrow base in the area of the red lip, which the labial artery supplies.

图2.83-1描绘了通过一卵圆形，贯穿下唇全层组织的切口来切除下唇肿瘤。在上唇外侧将取出1个三层皮瓣。该皮瓣蒂部延伸于上唇红中部。

Fig. 2.83-1 shows a tumor of the lower lip, which is removed by means of an oval excision through all thicknesses of the lower lip. In the region of the lateral upper lip, a three-layered flap is harvested. Its pedicle runs in the medial part of the lip vermilion.

如图2.83-2所示，将所形成的皮瓣扭转180°，覆盖下唇缺损部位，三层分层缝合。取皮瓣处可直接缝合来合并。第一期手术后14天可切断皮瓣蒂部并同时使上下唇的唇红/唇白边缘准确地整合在一起（图2.83-3）。

In Fig. 2.83-2 the flap is rotated at an angle of 180° into the lower lip defect and sutured in three layers. The donor region can be closed by direct approximation. Two weeks after the first operation (Fig. 2.83-3), the

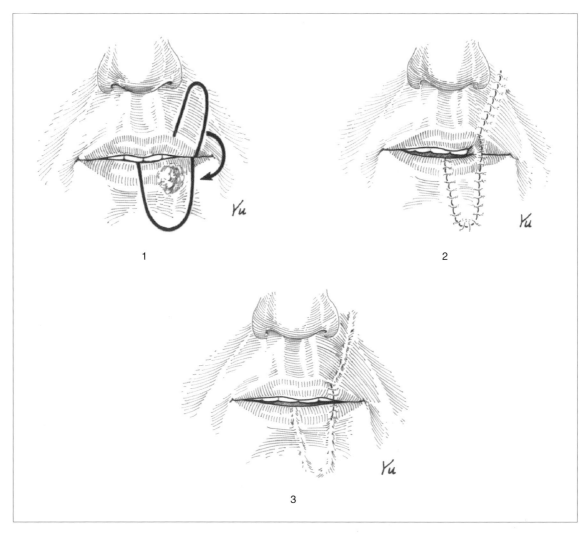

图2.83　ABBE方法

Fig. 2.83　Method according to ABBE

pedicle of the flap can be separated and, at the same time, the lip red/lip white border of both lips precisely reapproximated.

　　该方法的缺点在于必须进行二期手术。同时上唇的瘢痕不与鼻唇沟重合，而是与皮肤张力线稍有交叉。缺损修复仅适用于肿瘤不大的情况。

One drawback of this technique is that secondary operation is mandatory. Furthermore, the scar in the region of the upper lip does not lie in the axis of the nasolabial groove, but intersects the lines of minimal tension. Reconstruction of a defect via this method is feasible only if the tumor is not extensive.

ABBE皮瓣修复方法的矫正手术

　　在一期手术后3周的二期手术中，将切断皮瓣蒂部。同时唇红将覆盖一期手术中所涉及的口角（图2.84）。如图2.84－1所描绘的，皮瓣蒂部通过切口AB切开。切口BC沿瘢痕方向长1cm。第二条

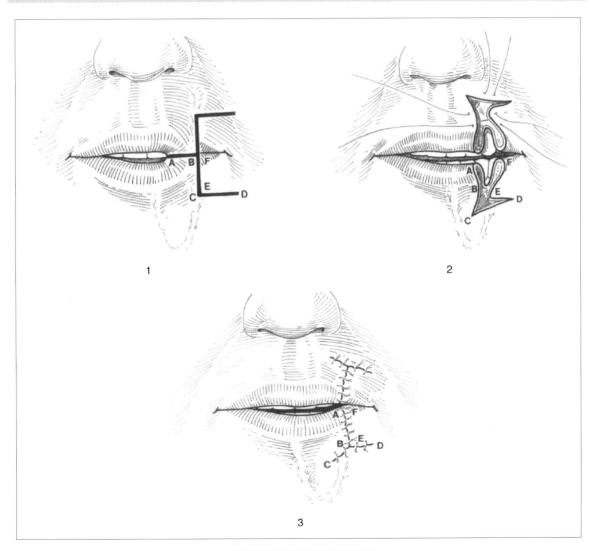

图2.84　根据ABBE矫正口角

Fig. 2.84　Mouth Angle Correction according to ABBE

切口沿水平方向，长度略大于1cm。在上唇区再作两条相同的切口。

Corrective Flap Plastic Surgery according to ABBE

In a second session, three weeks after the first operation, the flap pedicle is separated and the lip vermilion adapted to the mouth angle which was kept intact in the first operation (Fig. 2.84). In accordance with Fig. 2.84-1, the foot of the flap is divided by the incision AB. The incision BC is developed along the scar line from the first operation and is 1cm. in length. A third, horizontal incision, CD is slightly longer than 1 cm. Two analogous incisions are developed in the region of the upper lip.

图2.84-2描绘了切开后的状态。现在可进行切口边角的镶嵌缝合，缝合时唇红/唇白边缘对接于正确位置。由此形成点AF和BE段的边缘重合，从而将CD段从中间分开（图2.84-3）。

Fig. 2.84-2 shows the appearance after the incisions have been made. The edges of the incision are now approximated and sutured, taking care to adapt the red-white border of the lip with exactitude. This causes the points AF and BE to be on the edge and the line CD is reduced by half (Fig. 2.84-3).

ESTLAND手术（1872）

该方法适用于下唇外侧缺损的再造。

ESTLAND Operation (1872)

This method is indicated for reconstruction of lower lip defects in the lateral segment of the lower lip.

图2.85-1描绘了切除下唇肿瘤部位的切口以及用以形成位于上唇侧部的旋转皮瓣的切口。

Fig. 2.85-1 shows the excision of the tumorous segment of the lower lip and the incision made to form a rotation flap in the lateral part of the upper lip.

如图2.85-2中所示，该皮瓣通过旋转覆盖于所须修复的缺损处并已缝合。

In Fig. 2.85-2 this flap has been rotated and placed on the defect, then sutured.

图2.85-3描绘了二次手术后的状态，此时圆形的口角已被矫正。

Fig. 2.85-3 shows the appearance after the second operation, following correction of the rounded commissure.

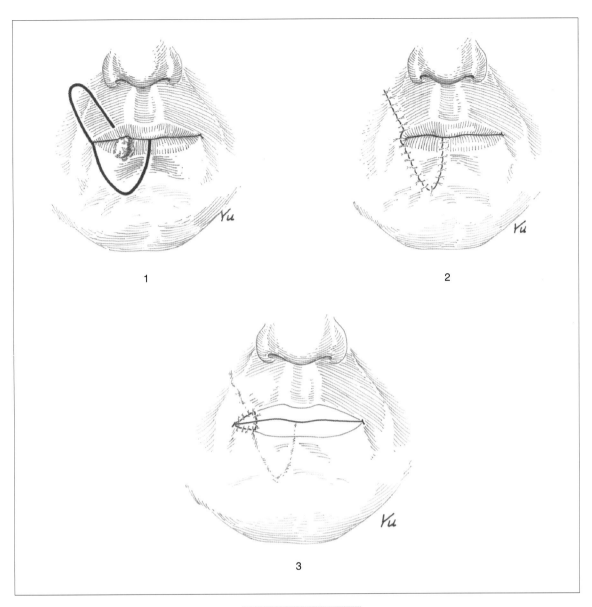

図2.85　ESTLAND方法

Fig. 2.85　Method according to ESTLAND

在切开新形成的圆形口角后,将在此区域切除一块三角形皮肤组织,将唇黏膜向侧面移动,同时所形成的缺损通过松动周边黏膜来覆盖。

在切开新形成的圆形口角后，将在此区域切除一块三角形皮肤组织，将唇黏膜向侧面移动，同时所形成的缺损通过松动周边黏膜来覆盖。

After the incision through the newly-formed, rounded commissure, a triangular piece of skin is excised from this region, the labial mucosa is shifted in a lateral direction and the resulting defect is covered by mobilized the adjacent mucosa.

改良的ESTLAND技术

此方法的适应证为下唇缺损大小为全部宽度的1/3～2/3。图2.86-1描绘了下唇部分的W形切口和用以形成改良ESTLAND皮瓣的切口。

Modified ESTLAND technique

This method is indicated when the lower lip defect involves between one and two thirds of the full breadth of the lower lip. The W-shaped excision of the lower lip segment and the line of incision for development of the modified Estland flap are shown in Fig. 2.86-1.

上唇区域的旋转皮瓣的宽度需要为下唇缺损宽度的一半。图2.86-2显示了所形成的下唇W形损伤，然后向尾部旋转的改良Estland皮瓣。

The length of the rotation flap in the region of the upper lip should correspond to one half of the breadth of the lower lip defect. Fig. 2.86-2 shows the created W-shaped defect of the lower lip and the caudally rotated modified Estlander flap.

图2.86-3显示了鼻唇沟皮区缺损直接缝合后的状态。

Fig. 2.86-3 shows the final result after direct approximation of the donor defect in the nasolabial region.

下唇中部的缺损可通过相同方式修复，状态见图2.86-4。

A defect situated in the mid-lower lip can be closed according to the same principle; this is illustrated in Fig. 2.86-4.

切除下唇中部1/3后，将在上唇再建一块矩形皮瓣，其与缺损宽度一半相符。另外，还需将含有口角区的连续的下唇部分向内侧推进与对侧的缺损部位边缘相拉近对位（图2.86-5）。

After excision of a median third of the lower lip, a rectangular flap is created from the upper lip, which corresponds to one half of the breadth of the defect. In addition, the pericommissural segment of the persistent lower lip is shifted medially and adapted to the defect edge on the opposite side (Fig. 2.86-5).

改良的ESTLAND皮瓣

该技术适用于楔形切口后形成的下唇楔形缺损。图2.87-1描绘了形成推进皮瓣和旋转皮瓣所需要的切口。口角区域的垂直切口向尾部延伸可使侧边下唇部分向中间推进。在鼻唇沟区域的切口显示用于再造手术典型的ESTLAND皮瓣。

Modified ESTLAND Flap

This technique is indicated when the lower lip defect is wedge-shaped. Fig. 2.87-1 shows the incision

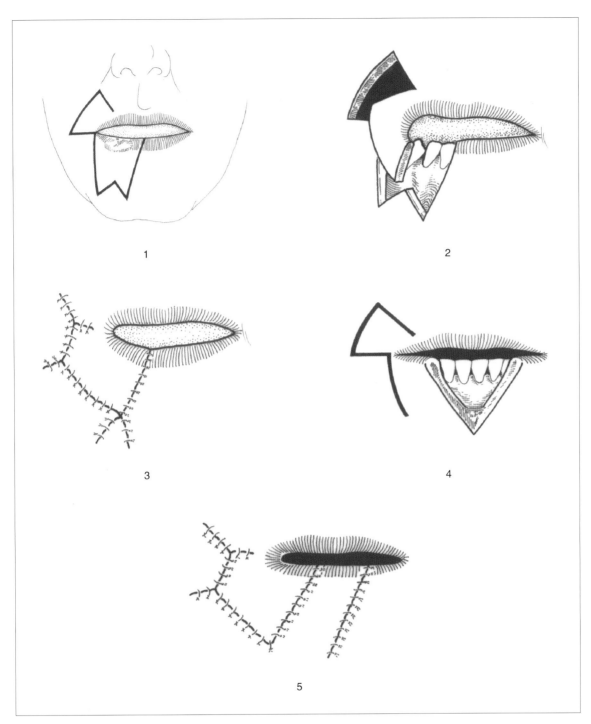

图2.86　改良的ESTLAND技术

Fig. 2.86　Modified ESTLAND technique

lines needed to create one advancement and one rotation flap. The vertical incision running caudally in the region of the oral commissure enables a medial shift of the lateral lower lip segment. In the nasolabial region, incision of a typical ESTLAND flap is indicated.

　　图2.87-2显示了下唇侧面部分水平推进覆盖缺损后的状态。图2.87-3显示了采用已形成的Estlander皮瓣来覆盖出现下唇侧面的缺损。

In Fig. 2.87-2, the lateral shift of the parietal segment of the lower lip into the original tumor defect has been performed. Closure of the lower lip defect—which now has become lateral—with the prepared Estlander flap is shown in Fig. 2.87-3.

Fig. 2.87-4 shows the end result after reconstruction. The right commissure is rounded.

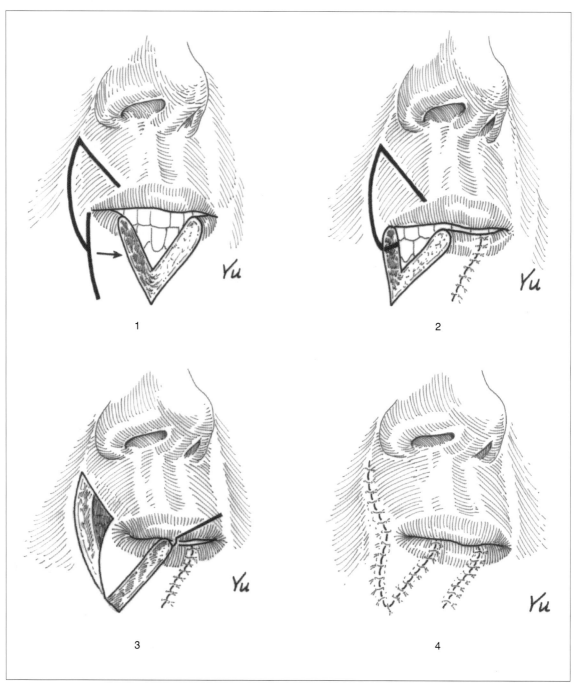

图2.87　改良的 ESTLAND皮瓣

Fig. 2.87   Modified ESTLAND Flap

GILLIES和MILLARD方法（1957）

该方法的适应证为下唇局部盒形缺损。

Method according to GILLIES and MILLARD (1957)

This method is indicated for box-shaped, partial lower lip defects.

图2.88-1图描绘了下唇中部的缺损以及由缺损边缘下部弧形向侧面上部延伸的松弛切口，设计两个Z形切口。在松动肌皮瓣后可将该瓣向下中间旋转并直接对位缝合。图2.88-2描绘了缺损修复后的形态以及运用的Z形成形术。

Fig. 2.88-1 shows the medial lower lip defect and a relaxing curvilinear incision which runs from the caudal edge of the defect in an upwardly lateral direction; in addition, it shows the creation of two Z-plasty incisions. The cutaneous muscle flap is mobilized and then rotated in a caudal-medial direction, then directly approximated and sutured. Fig. 2.88-2 shows the final result after closure of the defect and completed Z-plasty.

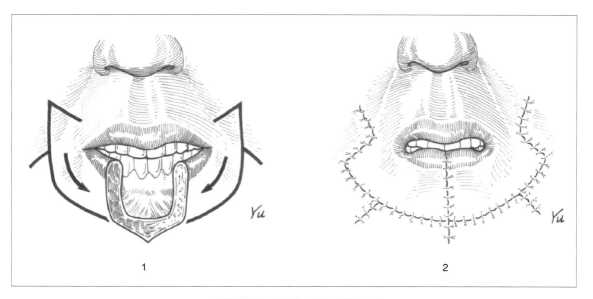

图2.88　GILLIES和MILLARD方法

Fig. 2.88　Method according to GILLIES and MILLARD

圆形口角的矫正（GILLIES和MILLARD，1957）

图2.89-1描绘了用于矫正圆形口角的切口线。口角侧面将切除一块三角形皮肤。该V形切口的下半弧形延伸至下唇红区域。由此形成一个蒂部位于上唇的黏膜瓣，小心仔细地将该瓣与口轮匝肌剥离。该瓣将被牵拉至先前形成的缺损处，即新的口角区域（图2.89-2）。

Correction of a rounded oral commissure (GILLIES and MILLARD, 1957)

Fig. 2.89-1 shows the incision lines for correction of a rounded mouth corner. A skin triangle is excised laterally to the region of the oral commissure. The inferior side of this V-shaped excision is developed in a curved shape into the vermilion area of the lower lip. This forms a mucosal flap which is pedicled in the upper lip. This flap is carefully separated from the underlying orbicularis oris muscle and set into in the previously created skin defect in the region of the new oral commissure (Fig. 2.89-2).

最后将完成下唇黏膜的剥离和相应的松动（图2.89-3）。在相应的松动后，将黏膜皮瓣向外旋转来覆盖下唇区域的黏膜缺损并直接用间断缝合法缝合（图2.89-4）。

Then, the lower lip mucosa is undercut and mobilized (Fig. 2.89-3). Following mobilization as outlined above, this mucosal flap can be rotated outwardly to cover/close the mucosal defect in the region of the lower lip and approximated by means of interrupted sutures (Fig. 2.89-4).

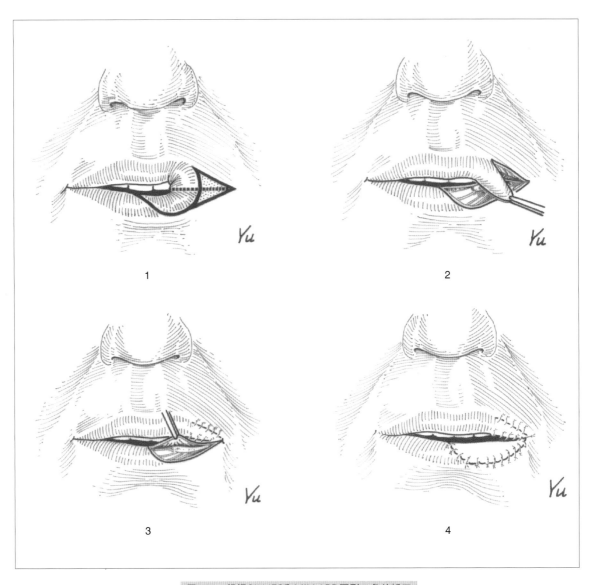

图2.89   根据GILLIES和MILLARD圆形口角的矫正

Fig. 2.89   Correction of a rounded oral commissure according to GILLIES and MILLARD

McGREGOR方法

该方法适用于下唇侧面一半缺损的再造。

Method according to McGREGOR

This method is indicated for reconstruction of a laterally situated defect involving one half of the lower lip.

图2.90-1描绘了下唇侧面部分的方形切除和形成近似直角的颊部皮瓣的切口线，供血由唇动脉来完成。该直角皮瓣的宽度与缺损处的扩张宽度相对应。

Fig. 2.90-1 shows the square excision of the lateral segment of the lower lip and the incision line for the development of a nearly square buccal flap. The flap is nourished by the labial artery. This square flap is as broad as the extension of the defect.

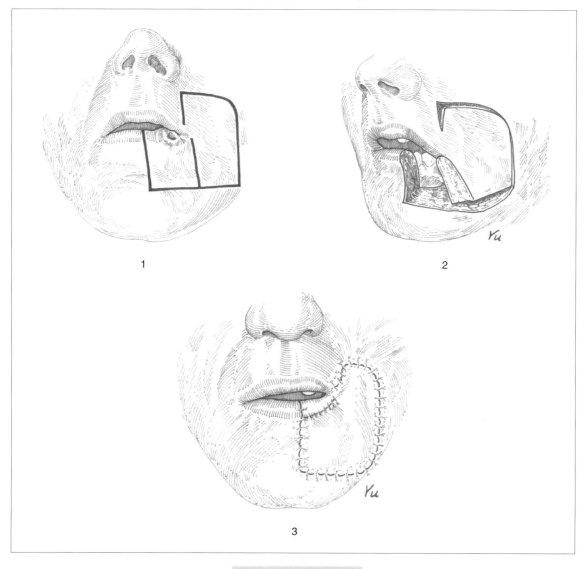

图2.90 McGREGOR方法

Fig. 2.90 Method according to McGREGOR

图2.90-2所示，将颊部皮瓣向中下方嵌入所要修复的缺损处并缝合。唇红将通过口腔前庭的黏膜来修复。

In Fig. 2.90-2, the buccal flap is shifted medially downwards into the defect and sutured. The lip vermilion is reconstructed from the oral vestibule by means of mobilized mucosa.

根据McGREGOR方法要优先选取舌皮瓣来修复唇红，因为采用黏膜推进皮瓣后的瘢痕愈合会导致收缩。

For reconstruction of the lip vermilion, McGREGOR prefers a tongue flap because the scar tissue from a mucosal advancement flap always causes the wound to contract upon healing.

图2.90-3显示了修复后的最终形态。

Fig. 2.90-3 shows the final state after reconstruction.

McGREGOR扇形皮瓣的改良

1984年NAKAJIMA等论述了改良的扇形皮瓣来再造下唇次全切除的矩形缺损。

Modification of McGREGOR's fan flap

In 1984, NAKAJIMA et al. described a modification of the fan-shaped flap used to reconstruct subtotal rectangular lower lip defects.

该皮瓣供血由位于上唇侧面含有唇动脉的狭长蒂部提供。

The entire flap is nourished by a narrow pedicle in the lateral region of the upper lip, which contains the labial artery.

图2.91-1描绘了下唇区域的矩形切除和用来形成扇形皮瓣的切口线。切口贯穿颊部全部三层组织并仔细保护面动脉。松动皮瓣后将其向下，向中间旋转并在中线处相会合。下唇红的重建采用前庭的黏膜（图2.91-2）。

Fig. 2.91-1 shows the rectangular excision in the region of the lower lip and the line of incision to create the fan-shaped flap. The incision traverses all thicknesses of the cheek, but the facial artery is carefully preserved. The flaps are mobilized and rotated in a downwardly medial direction, then approximated in the midline. The vermilion of the lower lip is reconstructed from the mucosa of the vestibule (Fig. 2.91-2).

最终形态参见图2.91-3。

The end state is shown in Fig. 2.91-3.

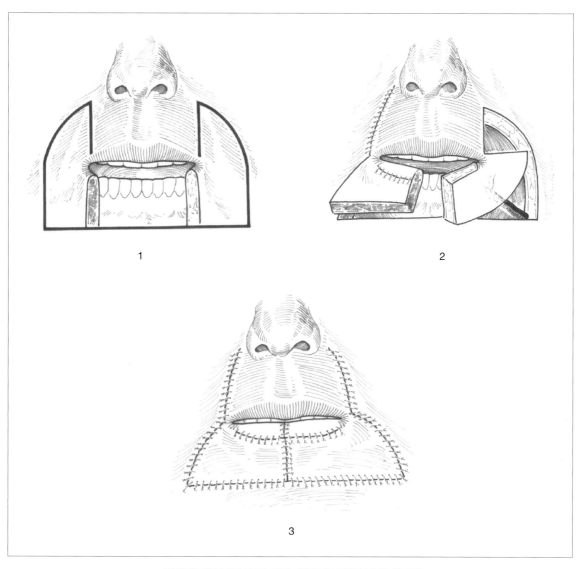

1

2

3

图2.91　根据NAKAJIMA et al.对McGREGOR方法改良

Fig. 2.91　Modification of the McGREGOR method according to NAKAJIMA et al

4.远位皮瓣

出于美观和功能顾虑，运用远位皮瓣技术来再造下唇是满意度最小的方法。只有当缺损位置达到超出下唇，同时也到达周边面颊区域和颏部区域，或者甚至达到下颌骨时才采用远位皮瓣。

4. Distant Flaps

Reconstruction of a lower lip defect by means of distant flaps is the least satisfactory method with respect to aesthetic and functional concerns. However, its indication should be considered, when the defect extends beyond the region of the lip to the adjacent buccal and mental regions, and possibly even the body of mandible is affected.

在上述大的缺损情况下，运用邻近皮瓣技术来修复下唇已经无法获得成功。

A defect of such an extension cannot be reconstructed by means of direct flap plastic surgery.

利用面罩式皮瓣（前额皮瓣）修复下唇

图2.92-1描绘了大的下唇肿瘤切除的切口以及形成双侧颞部桥形皮瓣。

Reconstruction of the lower lip by means of visor flaps (frontal flaps)

Fig. 2.92-1 shows the line of incision for excision of an extensive tumor of the lower lip and creation of a bi-temporal bridge flap.

图2.92-2所示将桥形皮瓣折起，额皮瓣供区通过一块游离皮片来覆盖。桥形皮瓣的供血由颞浅动脉分支来提供。

In Fig. 2.92-2, the bridge flap is folded and the donor area of the frontal flap is covered with a free split-thickness graft. The bridge flap is nourished by branches of the superficial temporal artery.

如图2.92-3中所描绘的，桥形皮瓣剩余的开放创面将构成一管状带蒂皮瓣（Rundstiellappen），从而避免创面裸露。带毛发部分的皮瓣宽度基本上要比不带毛发的皮瓣部分小1cm。带毛发部分和不带毛发部分的边缘采用间断缝合，同时避免产生空腔。用于替代黏膜的前额皮瓣的不带毛发的皮肤必须向外超出用于替代皮肤缺损的前额皮瓣的带毛发头皮，前者将用于再造唇红。外科手术后2~3周，该皮瓣将向下旋转180°覆盖缺损部位（图2.92-4）。

The sketch in Fig. 2.92-3 shows how the remaining open wound surface of the bridge flap is developed into a tubed pedicle flap in order to avoid open wound areas. As a rule, the hairy part is 1cm smaller in breadth than the hairless segment of the flap. The edges of the hairy and hairless flap areas are approximated by means of interrupted sutures, taking care to avoid cavitation. The hairless frontal skin used to replace the mucosa must project beyond the hairy scalp used to reconstruct the skin defect; the former is later used to reconstruct the vermilion of the lip. Two to three weeks after the first operation, the flap is rotated caudally by

180° and inset into the defect (Fig. 2.92-4).

缺损边缘须去掉表皮形成新鲜创面。沿带毛发-不带毛发皮肤的分界线作一条切口，将皮瓣切开有足够的缝隙，从而使带毛发皮肤可以形成唇外侧，不带毛发皮肤形成唇内侧（图2.92-5）。

The edge of the defect is deepithelialized and freshened. An incision is made along the borderline between hairy and hairless skin, and the flap is split along a certain distance, permitting the hairy skin to be on the exterior side of the lip and the hairless skin on the interior side (Fig. 2.92-5).

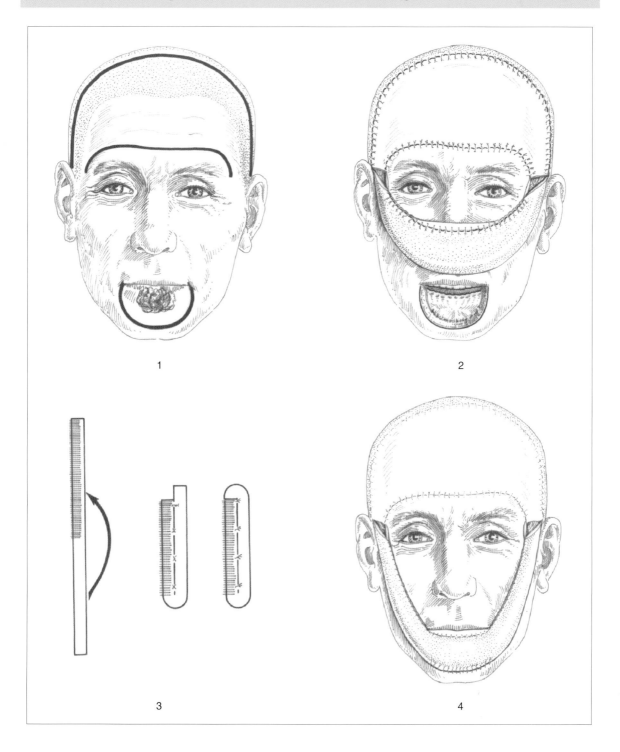

1

2

3

4

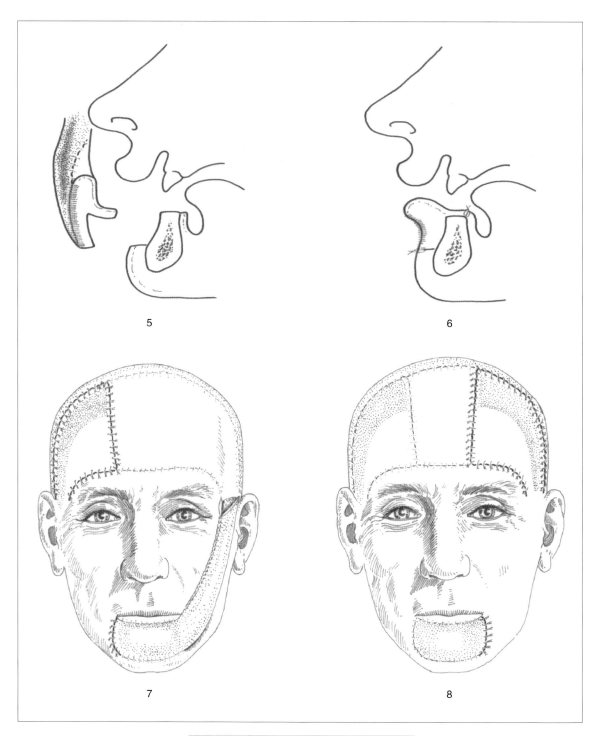

图2.92　利用双带蒂皮瓣（前额皮瓣）修复下唇

Fig. 2.92   Lower lip reconstruction by means of visor flaps (frontal flaps)

　　额皮瓣（不带毛发）游离的创面边缘将与缺损边缘的黏膜缝合，带毛发的创面边缘与皮肤缺损边缘缝合（图2.92-6）。

The free wound edge of the frontal flap (hairless) is sutured to the mucosa of the edge of the defect. The free wound edge of the frontal flap (hair) is sutured to the skin of the edge of the defect (Fig. 2.92-6).

再经过2周即可将供区相应位置切除相应宽度皮肤并将右侧皮瓣蒂部回迁至其原始位置，缝合。该三期手术后2周，可将左侧蒂部运用同样方法回迁（图2.92-7、图2.92-8）。

Two weeks later, the flap pedicle on the right side is shifted back and, after removal of a corresponding split-thickness skin graft, sutured into its original bed. Two weeks after this third operation, the pedicled flap on the left side is also shifted back as described above (Fig. 2.92-7 and Fig. 2.92-8).

Pharao技术

该技术由SOUSSALINE和KAUER于1977进行了描述。下唇的再造是采用1～2块折叠的胸三角皮瓣来完成（图2.93）。

"Pharao Technique"

This technique was described in 1977 by SOUSSALINE and KAUER. The lower lip is reconstructed by using one or two folded deltopectoral flaps (Fig. 2.93).

管状带蒂皮瓣

鉴于完整性的考虑，下唇再造还可通过管状带蒂皮瓣来完成。

Tubed Pedicle Flaps

For the sake of comprehensiveness, the possibility of reconstructing the lower lip with the aid of tubed pedicle flaps should be mentioned here.

如果供皮区来自全身，则主要会尝试取自胸、腹和肩部。基本上该方法要求多个手术步骤，同时无法在功能和美观上达到完全令人满意的下唇再造效果。

The donor site can be situated in any region of the body; the chest, stomach and shoulder are primarily used. In principle, these methods demand several operative steps and by no means allow for a functionally and aesthetically satisfactory reconstruction of the lower lip.

因此SCHUCHARDT将用管状带蒂皮瓣再造的唇区域表达为"自身材料假体"。

SCHUCHARDT called a lip region reconstructed with tubed pedicle flaps a "prostheses made of endogenous material".

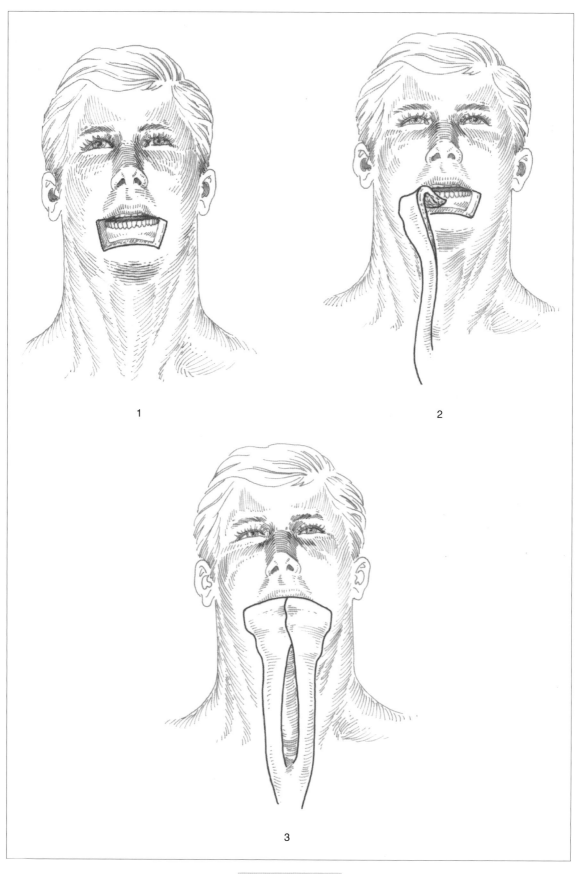

1

2

3

图2.93　Pharao技术

Fig. 2.93　"Pharao Technique"

第**3**章

Chapter 3

我的下唇再造技术
My Method of Lower Lip Reconstruction

1. 手术技术

图3.1显示下唇肿瘤在确保安全距离的前提下，通过心形切口，贯穿全层组织进行切除。

1. Operative Technique

Fig. 3.1 shows a tumor in the lower lip that is to be excised with a safety margin using a heart-shaped incision through all layers of the lower lip.

点J位于心形切口的顶点。虚线A-B表示一松弛切口，从嘴角水平向侧边延伸，其长度略长于缺损宽度的一半。这可保证形成丰满完整的下唇。虚线D-C须略带弧形经过B点向下并与鼻唇沟重叠。B-C段长约1.5cm。D-E长度约为D-A段的一半并与A-B垂直。A-B-G区域的皮肤之后将由于形成下唇红而切除。

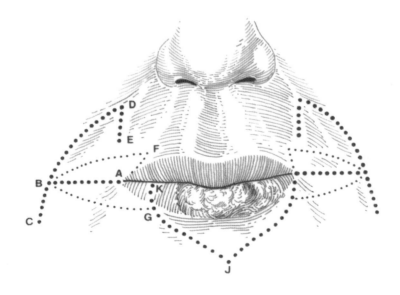

图3.1

Fig. 3.1

Point J is at the apex of the heart-shaped incision. The dotted horizontal line A−B shows a relieving incision running laterally from the corner of the mouth. The line A−B is slightly longer than half the width of the surgical defect. This allows for the reconstruction of a full voluminous lower lip. The dotted line D, C should be slightly curved and overlap the nasolabial fold in the caudal direction by crossing B. The line B−C is about 1.5 cm long. D−E runs perpendicular to A−B and has a length corresponding to one-half of the distance D, A. The skin in A−B−G will later be excised for the reconstruction of the lower lip vermilion.

虚线B−F−A所对应的黏膜皮瓣将之后用于再造下唇。相同的切口也在对边做出。图3.2显示下唇肿瘤切除后的形态。

The corresponding mucous membrane flap for later reconstruction is consistent with the dotted line B-F-A. The same incisions are performed on the opposite side of the mouth. In Fig. 3.2 the excision of the tumor in the lower lip has been performed.

图3.3显示水平方向的松弛切口A−B。然后作皮肤B−C的切口。剥离获得的A−B−C皮肤瓣，其下的表情肌（口轮匝肌、颧大肌、笑肌、口角降肌）将被显示出来。

Fig. 3.3 shows the horizontal relieving incisions A-B, followed by the incision of the skin from B to C. The resulting skin flap A-B-C is mobilized, exposing the underlying mimic muscles (orbicularis oris, zygomaticus major, risorius, depressor anguli oris).

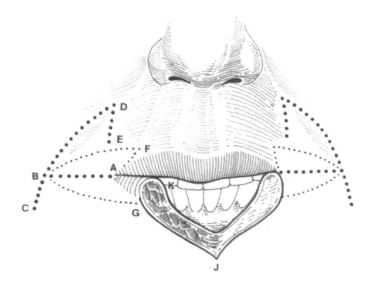

图3.2

Fig. 3.2

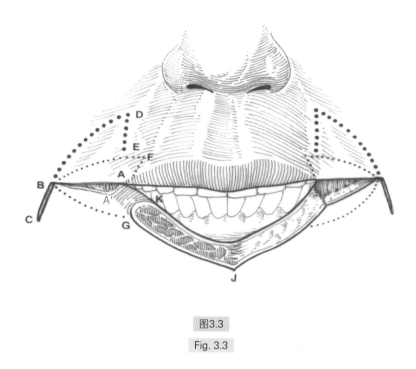

图3.3

Fig. 3.3

　　图3.4描绘了对应于外侧虚线A−F−B−C来切割内侧黏膜瓣A′−F′−B′−C′。该黏膜瓣将用于修复下唇红。

Fig. 3.4 shows the incision of the inner mucous membrane flap A′ -F′ -B′ -C′ that corresponds to the outer discontinuous line A-F-B-C. This mucous membrane flap serves to reconstruct the lower lip vermilion.

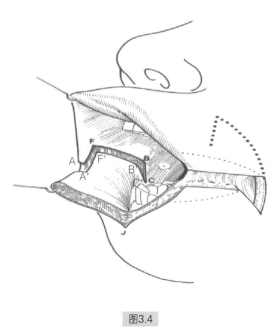

图3.4

Fig. 3.4

图3.5所示，口角处口轮匝肌的内侧部分将被切开，外侧肌肉部分受到保护。在部分切开近口角的口轮匝肌后，沿虚线HI肌肉纤维方向分离口轮匝肌。最终将C-B-H-I区域的皮肤与其下方的肌肉剖离。从而在内侧部分（I-H-K-J）获得一个复合的肌肉–皮肤瓣，在外侧部分（C-B′-H-I）获得一个纯皮肤皮瓣。

　　Fig. 3.5 shows that the medial part of the auricularis oris is cut at the corner of the mouth, the lateral part of the muscle is kept intact. After partial transection of the part of the orbicularis close to the commissure, the orbicularis is split along the line H−I, following the grain of the muscle. Corresponding to the area C−B′−H−I, the skin is dissected and mobilized from the underlying muscle. The result is a composite muscle and skin flap in the medial area (I−H−K−J) and a pure skin flap in the lateral area (C−B′−H−I).

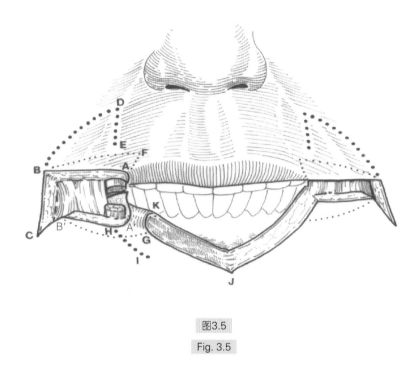

图3.5

Fig. 3.5

　　图3.6描绘了重建后的下唇。皮瓣C-B′-K-J与对侧皮瓣相缝合。图中还可见下唇断端的双侧位移。

　　Fig. 3.6 shows the reconstructed lower lip. The flap C−B′ − K−J is sutured to its corresponding flap on the opposite site. The bilateral dislocation of the lower lip stumps is shown in Fig. 3.6.

　　图3.7显示了对应于线段A-B，B-D，和D-E位于鼻唇区域的辅助切口。通过该辅助切口获得的皮肤瓣A-B-D′-E将被移动并通过旋转向后拉伸。从而使下唇区域侧边的缺损可以缝合（图3.8）。

Fig. 3.7 shows auxiliary incisions in the nasolabial area, corresponding to line A−B, B−D and D−E. A triangular skin flap A−B − D′ −E is mobilized and rotated downwards. In this way, the defect on both sides of the lateral lower lip area can be sutured (Fig. 3.8).

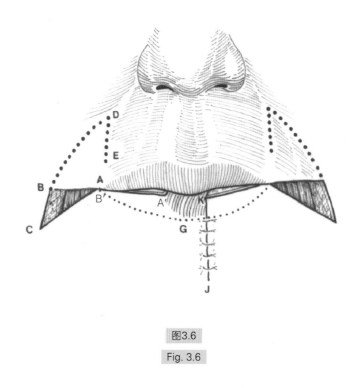

图3.6

Fig. 3.6

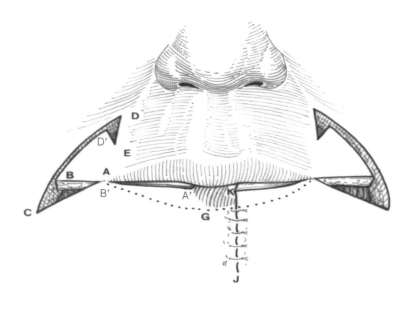

图3.7

Fig. 3.7

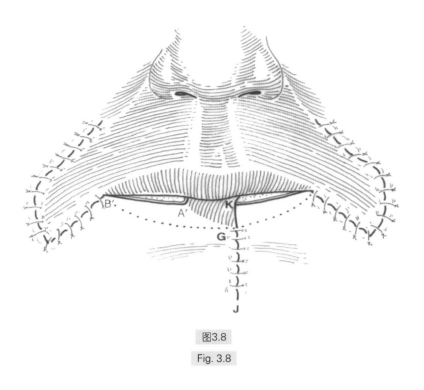

图3.8

Fig. 3.8

　　在切除A′-B′-G区域的皮肤后（图3.8），将内侧黏膜瓣用Gillies单钩向外旋转并与再造的下唇白缝合。在口腔前庭所形成的黏膜缺损可直接愈合（图3.9）。

After excision of the skin in A′-B′-G the inner flap of the mucous membrane is rotated out-wards with a Gillies skin hook and sutured to the reconstructed lower lip white (Fig. 3.8). The resulting defects of the mucous membrane in the oral vestibule can be approximated directly (Fig. 3.9).

　　图3.10描绘了修复后的缝合线。

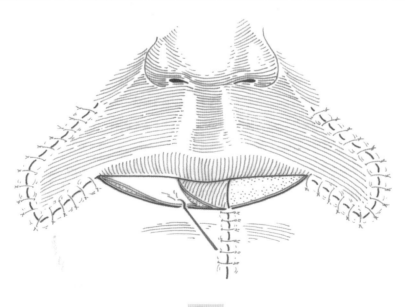

图3.9

Fig. 3.9

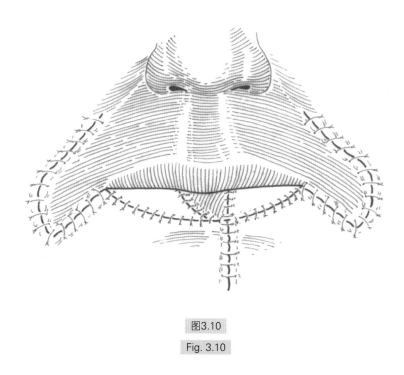

图3.10

Fig. 3.10

Fig. 3.10 shows the suture line after completion of the reconstruction.

2. 手术中的要点以及术后护理的要点

为了使下唇切除及重建的手术进展顺利并达到良好的术后效果，需注意以下几点。

2. Specifics during Operation and Postoperative Treatment

To achieve favorable progress of the operation and a satisfactory postoperative result of the lower lip resection with subsequent reconstruction, the following points are to be considered.

（1）切口的选择

如果下唇切除的部分不超过下唇1/3，下唇肿瘤切除后形成的缺损还是容易闭合的。如果切除后缺损为1/3～1/2下唇宽度，则建议单侧运用所介绍的方法。如果必须切除的部分超过下唇1/2，则B点须低于连线A－B大约3mm。AB表示口裂的水平延长线。另外点C须向中间偏移大约3mm。通过这些更改，可使再造达到更佳的效果。

(1) Type of Incision

After excision of the tumor of the lower lip, the newly formed defect can be closed easily if not more than one-third of the lower lip had to be excised. If the defect is equivalent to 1/3 to 1/2 of the width of the lower lip, the introduced method is recommended unilaterally. If more than half of the lower lip is to be resected, point B is to be located about 3 mm below the connecting line A-B which represents the horizontal extension of the oral fissure. Furthermore, point C is to be moved medially by about 3 mm. By this modified type of incision the reconstruction result will be more favorable.

如果切除后的缺损位于下唇中间，须在两边做切口；如果切除后的缺损覆盖整个下唇，则切口A-B的长度必须略大于下唇宽度的一半。

If the resection defect is situated in the center of the lower lip, the type of incision is to be applied on both sides; if the resection defect covers the entire lower lip, the length of the incision A-B must be larger than half of the width of the lower lip.

（2）形成皮瓣

当旋转皮瓣和推进皮瓣时，必须保证面神经不受损伤。面动脉的血管供应没有必要特别注意，因为即使有所损伤，也不会对皮瓣供血造成干扰。当皮下脂肪过厚时，须进行足够的削减。

(2) Formation of the Flap

The branches of nervus facialis must not be injured when mobilizing the rotational flap and advancement flap. The vascular supply by arteria facialis does not have to be considered in particular as the blood supply of the flap will not be disrupted if it is injured. In the case of excessive subcutaneous fat, it is to be reduced sufficiently.

（3）再造唇红

修复唇红的黏膜面积须足够大。基于此目的，用两根针向口腔方向垂直通过F点、B点和颊软组织。两根针之间颊部黏膜区域可选取一条略带弧形的切口线。作一条2mm高的黏膜切口，从而形成一块大的用于修复唇红的黏膜瓣。

(3) Reconstruction of the Lip Vermilion

The mucous membrane for the reconstruction of the lip vermilion is to be made available in sufficient quantity. For this purpose, two cannulae are inserted vertically through points F, B and the buccal soft tissue in oral direction. Between the two cannulae, a slightly curved type of incision in the buccal soft tissue area is to be preferred. If the incision in the mucous membrane is performed 2 mm higher, a larger mucous membrane flap for the reconstruction of the lip vermilion can be formed.

（4）保护表情肌肉组织

由于嘴角区域相对皮下组织较少，厚度为2~3mm，与肌肉组织相互粘连，形成皮瓣必须小心。通过使用15号或11号手术刀片容易看到表情肌肉组织，然后口轮匝肌内侧半将被切开。肌肉外侧部分将被保护隔离，以确保口轮匝肌功能完全。

(4) Conservation of the Mimic Muscles

As there is relatively little subcutaneous tissue around the corner of the mouth—it is only about 2–3 mm thick—that is conjoined to the muscles, caution is advised when forming the flap. Using a scalpel blade No. 15 or 11, the mimic muscles are displayed easily. The medial half of orbicularis oris is divided afterwards. The lateral part of the muscle is conserved to preserve the function of the orbicular muscle.

（5）闭合黏膜

当形成红唇时，将颊部黏膜向外牵拉并使用纤细的缝合线（Prolene 5.0）与重建的下唇缝合。由于嘴角区域的组织承受大部分的张力，为了保证缝合力度，故进行两道皮下缝合。创面的其他部分采用Prolene线3.0缝合。没有必要置入胶皮条。

(5) Sealing of the Mucous Membrane

For the reconstruction of the lower lip vermilion, the buccal mucous membrane is flipped outwardly and is sutured to the skin of the reconstructed lower lip with thin suture material (Prolene 5.0). As the tissue around the commissure is mostly tense, two subcutaneous sutures are performed to support the main suture. The remaining part of the wound is closed with Prolene 3.0. A rubber drain is not required.

（6）术后护理

术后建议在创面使用抗生素药膏。另外可以使用压力绷带和冰块。手术前后短期高剂量，预防使用抗生素就足够了。

(6) Postoperative Treatment

The application of an antibiotic ointment to the wound is recommended. Additionally, an adhesive pressure bandage and ice are to be applied. A short-term high-dosed perioperative antibiotic prophylaxis is sufficient.

第 **4** 章

Chapter 4

病例说明

Case Descriptions

病例1

病史

53岁的患者3个月前开始在下唇观察到一缓慢生长的肿瘤，作为治疗的主要手段药物治疗未取得好效果。患者称有时自发性出血，由于这个原因患者被初步诊断为下唇癌并转入我院。

Case 1

Anamnesis

The 53-year-old patient has been observing a slowly growing swelling at the lower lip for 3 months. A primarily conducted drug treatment was unsuccessful. The patient reported spontaneous hemorrhage every now and then. On this account, the patient was referred to our clinic with the tentative diagnosis "carcinoma of the lower lip".

检查结果

下唇红与唇白交界处的中心区域发现一个向正中左侧扩展的下唇癌变，中心存在结痂的溃疡，周边厚且呈凸起状。浸润生长的肿瘤面积为3cm×1.5cm。触诊检查颈部淋巴结，发现颏下左侧一个肿大的、触痛易推动的淋巴结。

Findings

A tumorous mutation is visible on the median area of the lower lip vermilion/white border, extending towards left paramedian. Central ulcerations with scabbing and raised rims. The diameter of the growing infiltrative tumor was 3cm × 1.5cm. The palpatory examination of the cervical lymph node showed an enlarged, pressure indolent and easily relocatable lymph node on the submandibular left.

在快速病理切片初步诊断为"鳞状上皮细胞癌"后，先施行舌骨上淋巴结清除术并切除肿瘤后运用上述方法进行再造。

After histological rapid section confirmation of the tentative diagnosis "squamous cell carcinoma", a suprahyoid lymphadenectomy and resection of the tumor and reconstruction according to the method outlined above were performed.

术后8.5个月后状态良好，无复发迹象。唇形及功能令人非常满意（图4.1.1～图4.1.13）。

8.5 months postoperative the condition was nonirritated. It showed no indication of tumor recurrence. The form and function of the lip were highly satisfactory (Fig. 4.1.1 to Fig. 4.1.13).

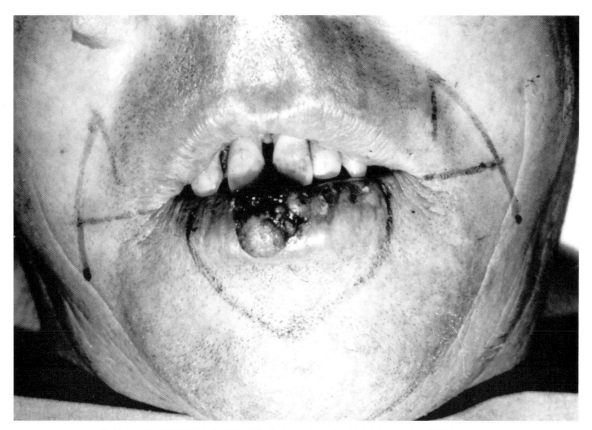

图4.1.1 有肿瘤的下唇行次全切除的切口线，鼻唇沟区域与口裂延长区域的辅助切口标记

Fig. 4.1.1 Incision lines for the subtotal removal of the tumor-bearing lower lip. Markings of auxiliary incisions in the nasolabial area and in the extension of the oral fissure

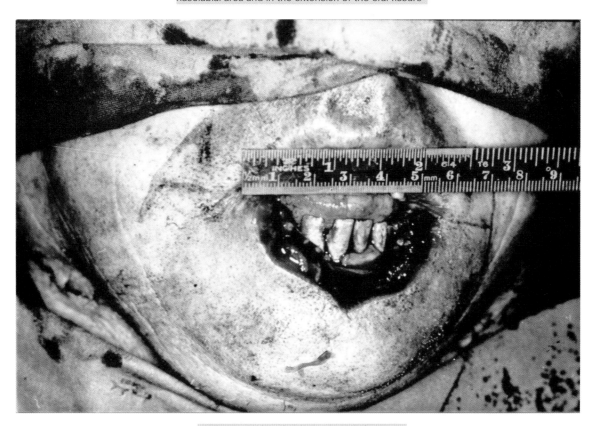

图4.1.2 肿瘤切除后状态，缺损宽度为5cm

Fig. 4.1.2 Condition after removal of the tumor. The defect width is 5cm

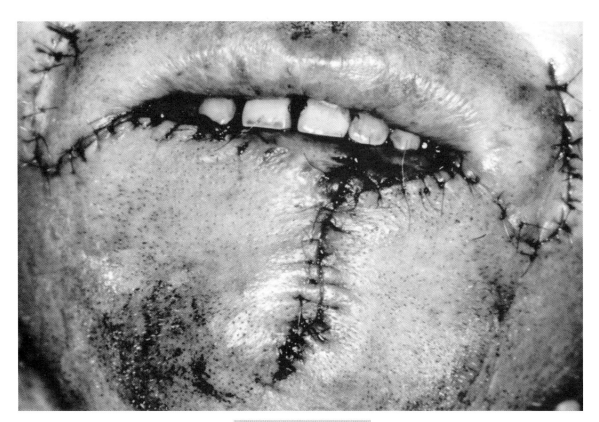

图4.1.3　下唇再造术后状态

Fig. 4.1.3　Condition after reconstruction of the lower lip

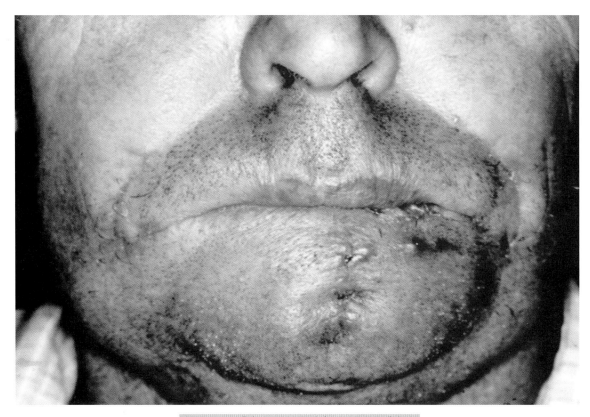

图4.1.4　闭嘴表现，下唇再造术后20天的闭嘴表现

Fig. 4.1.4　Mouth closed 20 days postoperative after lower lip reconstruction

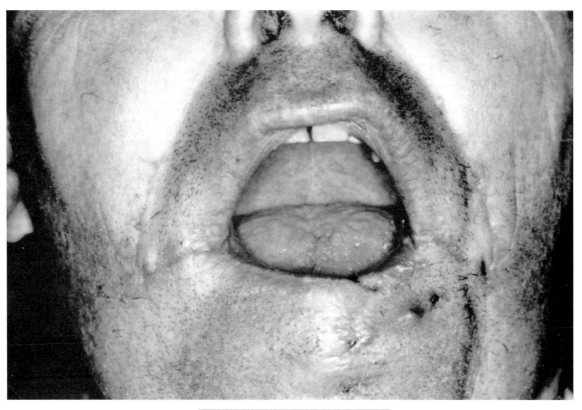

图4.1.5　开口表现，下唇再造术后20天

Fig. 4.1.5　Mouth opened 20 days postoperative after lower lip reconstruction

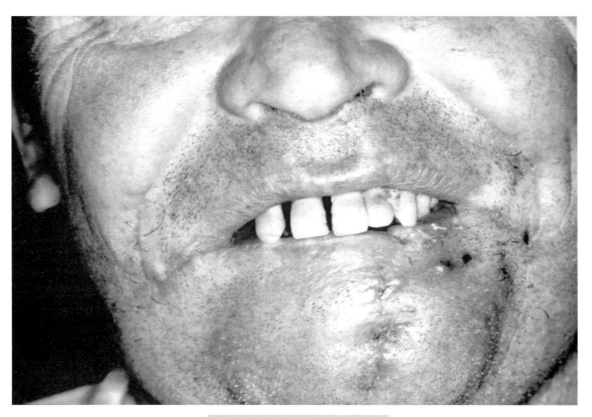

图4.1.6　术后20天微笑时表情肌功能

Fig. 4.1.6　Mimic function when laughing 20 days postoperative

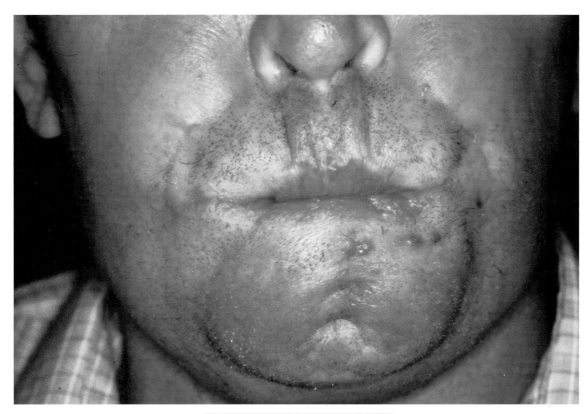

图4.1.7 术后20天噘嘴时口轮匝肌功能

Fig. 4.1.7 Function of orbicularis oris when pursing the lips 20 days postoperative

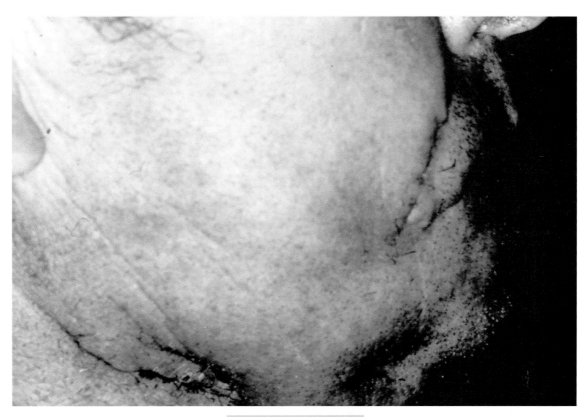

图4.1.8 口周区域的侧面观

Fig. 4.1.8 Profile shot of the perioral region

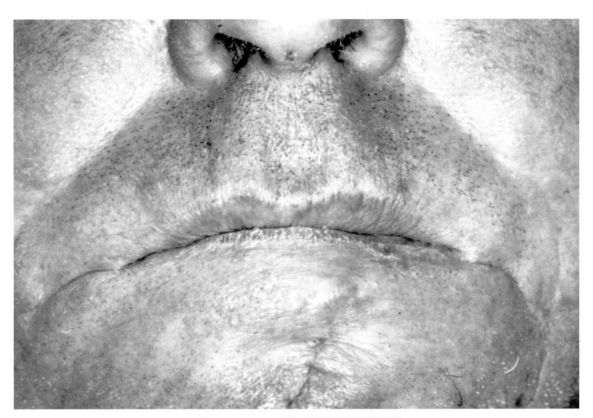

图4.1.9　下唇再造术后8.5个月的闭嘴表现

Fig. 4.1.9　Mouth closed 8.5 months postoperative after lower lip reconstruction

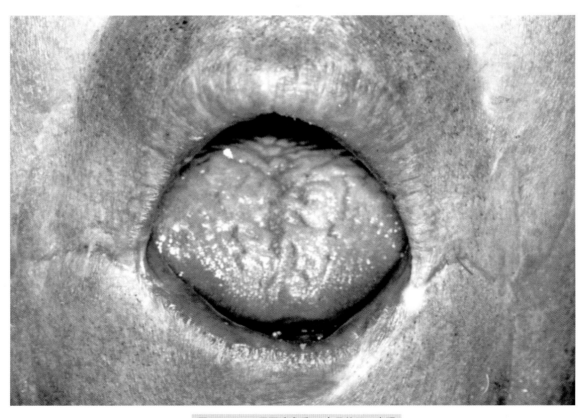

图4.1.10　下唇再造术后8.5个月的开口表现

Fig. 4.1.10　Mouth opened 8.5 months postoperative after reconstruction of the lower lip

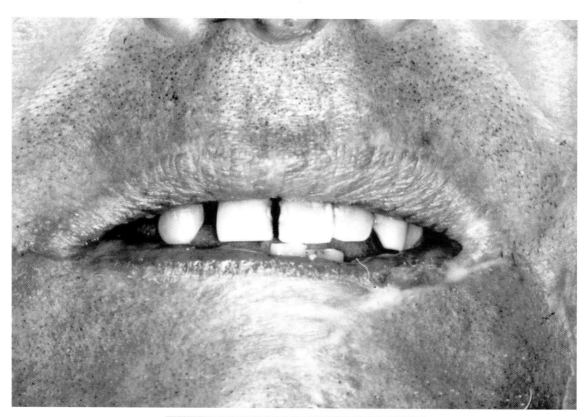

图4.1.11　下唇再造术后8.5个月的"露齿"时的唇功能

Fig. 4.1.11　Lip function when "showing teeth", 8.5 months after reconstruction of the lower lip

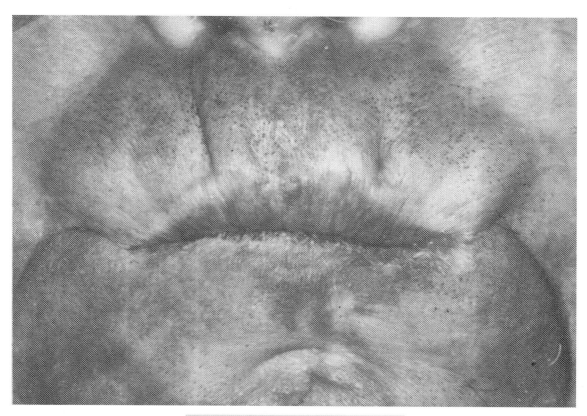

图4.1.12　术后8.5个月的抿嘴时口轮匝肌功能

Fig. 4.1.12　Function of orbicularis oris when pursing the lips 8.5 months postoperative

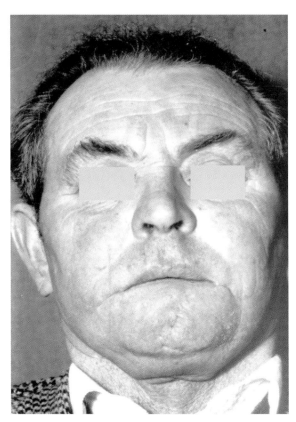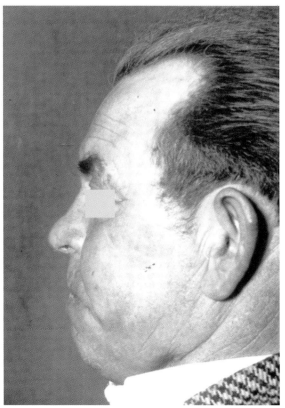

图4.1.13　下唇次全切除术后8.5个月的正、侧面观

Fig. 4.1.13　En face and profile 8.5 months postoperative after reconstruction of the subtotal lower lip

病例2

病史

55岁的患者3个月前开始在下唇左侧观察到反复发作的溃疡，据患者自己描述，其间偶尔愈合但又复发。经咨询家庭医生后，初诊为"下唇癌"并转入我院。

Case 2

Anamnesis

The 55-year-old patient has been observing a recurring ulcer on the left lower lip for three months that, according to the patient, has healed and recurred spontaneously multiple times. After consultation of the general practitioner the patient was referred to our clinic with the tentative diagnosis "carcinoma of the lower lip".

在下唇左侧发现一个直径1.5cm的肿瘤，中间溃疡，周边凸起。肉眼所见有0.5cm的浸润范围。淋巴循环系统检查发现颏下左侧有可触及的淋巴结。

The left part of the lower lip showed a tumor with a diameter of 1.5 cm with central ulceration and raised rims. Macroscopically extended infiltration of 0.5 cm was visible. The examination of the effluent lymphatic drainage system showed a palpable relocatable lymph node on the submandibular left.

在快速病理切片初步诊断为"鳞状上皮细胞癌"后，先施行左侧舌骨上淋巴结清除术，并切除肿瘤后运用上述方法进行再造术。

After preoperative histological rapid section confirmation of the tentative diagnose "squamous cell carcinoma" a suprahyoid lymphadenectomy on the left side and subsequent tumor resection as well as reconstruction of the lower lip according to the method outlined above were performed.

该病例术后也展现出了功能和美观上令人非常满意的效果（图4.2.1～图4.2.5）。

Postoperatively, the aesthetic and functional result was highly satisfactory as well (Fig. 4.2.1 to Fig. 4.2.5).

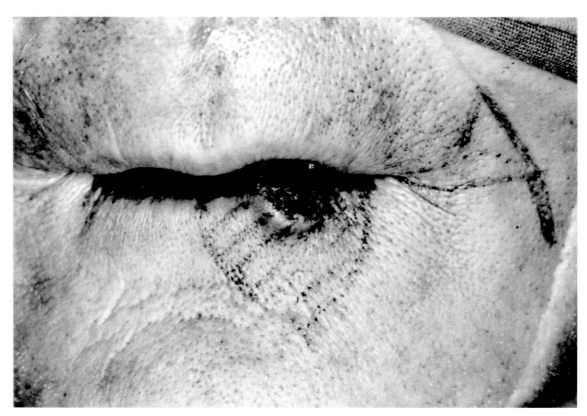

图4.2.1　显示下唇左侧肿瘤并在上面标记了切除肿瘤的心形切口和左侧辅助切口

Fig. 4.2.1　shows the tumor on the left lateral lower lip with markings for a heart–shaped type of incision for the excision of the tumor and auxiliary incision on the left side

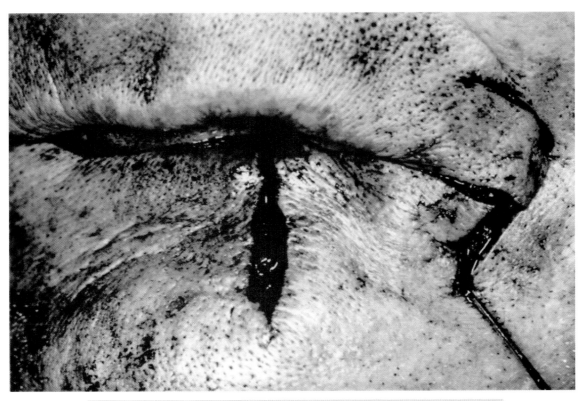

图4.2.2　肿瘤切除后状态，周边面颊软组织向中间推进并将皮瓣自鼻唇区域旋转至缺损处

Fig. 4.2.2　Condition after excision of the tumor, advancement of the adjoining buccal soft tissue towards medial and rotation of the flap from the nasolabial region into the defect

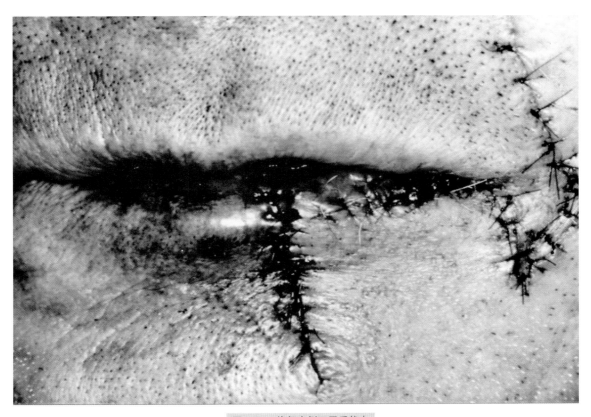

图4.2.3　修复半侧下唇后状态

Fig. 4.2.3　Condition after reconstruction of half of the lower lip

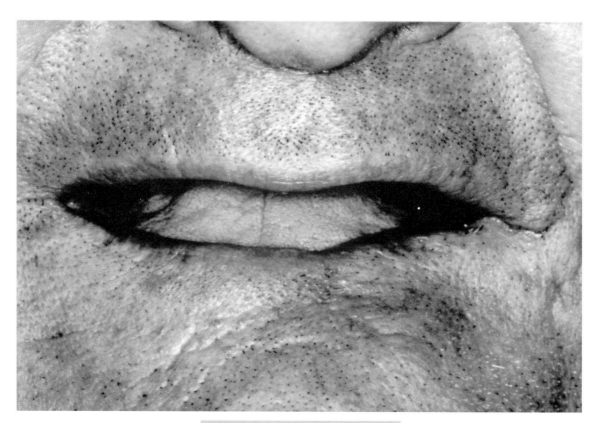

图4.2.4　术后30天临床功能（微笑）图片

Fig. 4.2.4　Clinical picture of function (laughing) 30 days postoperative

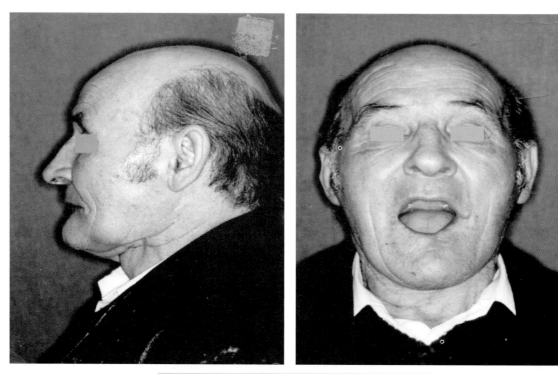

图4.2.5　下唇左侧半缺损再造术后30天，侧面观，开口位

Fig. 4.2.5　Profile and mouth opening 30 days postoperative after reconstruction of a defect that included half of the width of the lower lip on the left side

病例3

病史

70岁男性患者3个月前开始发现下唇出现反复发作，并有时疼痛的泛红和溃疡。家庭医生实施的药膏疗法无疗效。咨询牙医后转入皮肤科进行病理检查。基于病理结论为"鳞状上皮细胞癌"，介绍患者到Erlangen大学口腔颌面外科医院，患者25年前就已经因下唇癌接受过放射治疗。

Case 3

Anamnesis

A 70-year-old man has been noticing a recurring and partly painful redness and ulceration of the lower lip for 3 months. An ointment therapy conducted by the general practitioner was unsuccessful. Only after consultation of a dentist, the patient was referred to a dermatologist who conducted a sample collection. Based on the histological result "squamous cell carcinoma", the patient was referred to the Clinic for Maxillofacial Surgery Erlangen. 25 years earlier, the patient had been treated with radiation therapy for a carcinoma of the lower lip.

口腔外检查

下唇中间角质化肿瘤2cm×1cm。浸润深度0.5cm；无溃疡，无特殊感染。下颌下两侧触摸无淋巴结。除此无其他显著发现。1984年12月28日施行双侧舌骨上淋巴结清除术，保证安全距离的前提下，切除肿瘤。下唇中间的缺损为下唇宽度一半。最终对其采用上述方法再造下唇，唇形和功能非常满意（图4.3.1～图4.3.5）。

Extraoral findings:

Keratinizing tumor with the size of 2cm × 1cm in the center of the lower lip. Extension depth 0.5 cm; no ulceration, no superinfection. No palpable lymph node on either side submandibular. Otherwise without further pathological findings. On December, 28th 1984, the tumor was excised with a safety margin after suprahyoid lymphadenectomy on both sides. The defect of the medial lower lip was equal to half of the lower lip width and was followed by a lower lip reconstruction using the method outlined above. The form and the function of the lip are highly satisfactory (Fig. 4.3.1 to Fig. 4.3.5).

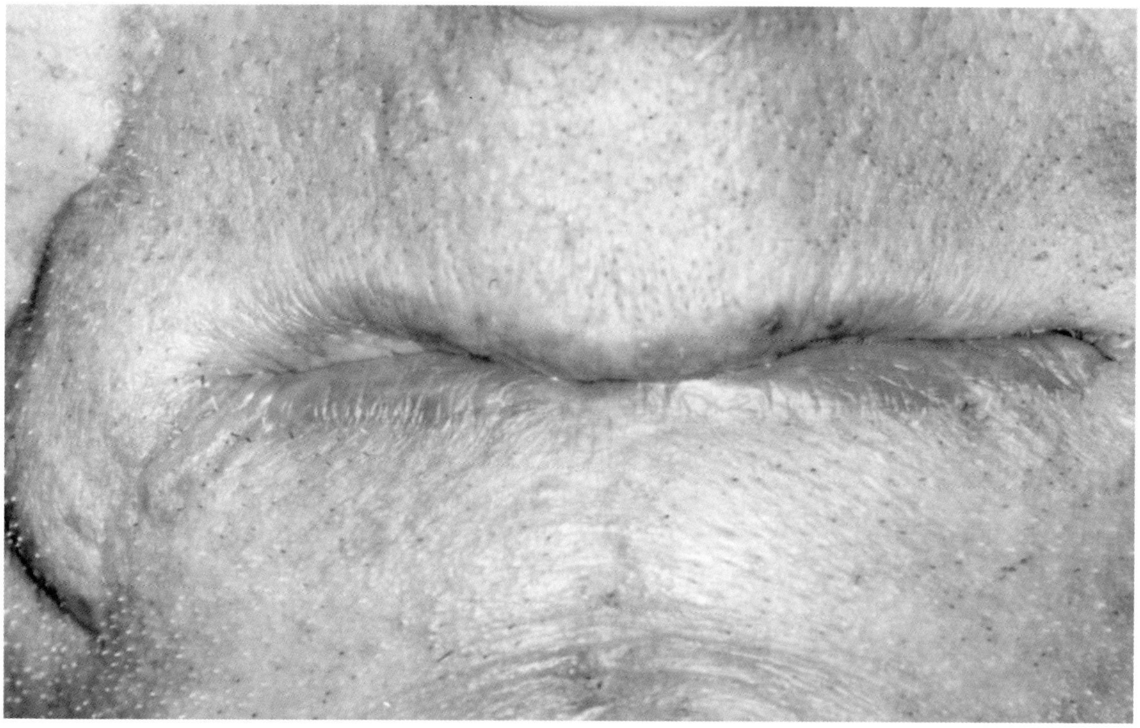

图4.3.1 下唇中间再造术后40天闭嘴状

Fig. 4.3.1 Mouth closed 40 days postoperative after reconstruction of the center of the lower lip

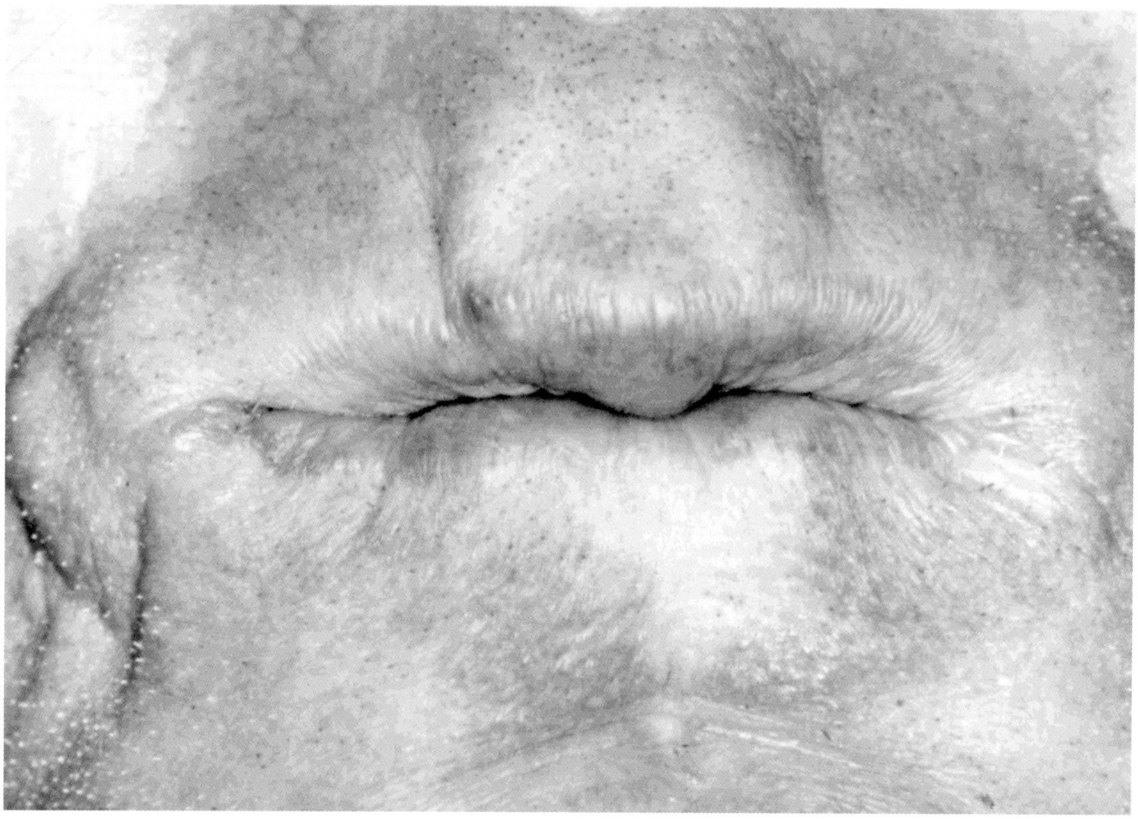

图4.3.2 修复后噘嘴时唇功能

Fig. 4.3.2 Function of the reconstructed lip when pursing the lips

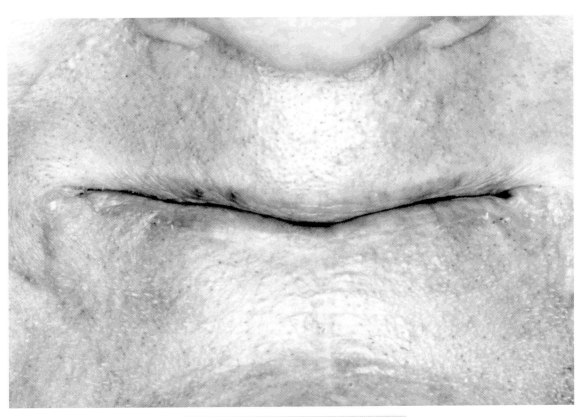

图4.3.3　微笑时表情功能，下唇再造术后40天

Fig. 4.3.3　Mimic function when laughing 40 days postoperative after lower lip reconstruction

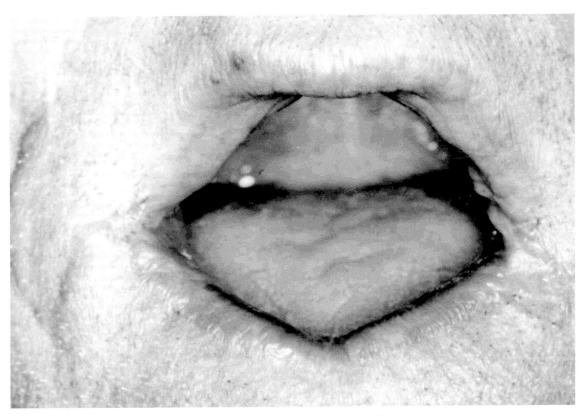

图4.3.4　下唇再造术后40天开口状

Fig. 4.3.4　Mouth opened 40 days postoperative after lower lip reconstruction

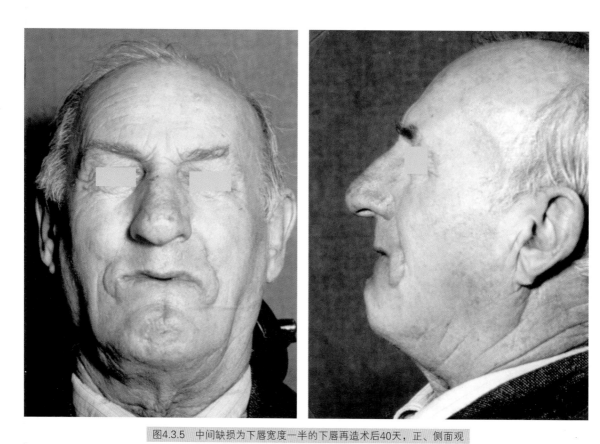

图4.3.5　中间缺损为下唇宽度一半的下唇再造术后40天，正、侧面观

Fig. 4.3.5　En face and profile 40 days postoperative after reconstruction of a medial defect covering half of the width of the lower lip

第 **5** 章

Chapter 5

讨论

Discussion

本书介绍了一种自己创新的肌功能改进的下唇再造新技术。在1984年4月至1985年2月期间，在Erlangen–Nuremberg大学口腔颌面外科门诊医院共为12位下唇肿瘤患者进行了手术。

This paper presents a new, self-developed, myofunctional, modified technique for reconstruction of the lower lip. At large, 12 patients with lower lip tumors were operated on at the Clinic and Policlinic for Maxillofacial Surgery Erlangen-Nuremberg between April 1984 and February 1985.

其中3位男性患者和1位女性患者年龄在53～76岁之间，通过GILLIES和McGREGOR方法成功完成了再造。对于其余8名男性患者采用了本文中介绍的肌功能重建方法。所有患者均为下唇鳞状上皮细胞癌。最年轻的患者为39岁，最年长患者为76岁。在患者中还有一位25年前就由于鳞状上皮细胞癌而经过放射治疗的患者。4名患者采用了双侧皮瓣推进的方式。另外4名患者则只需采用单侧旋转推进皮瓣这一术式。

For three male and one female patient between 53 and 76 years of age, the reconstructions were performed using the method of GILLIES and McGREGOR. The outlined myofunctional reconstruction method was performed on eight additional male patients. All patients were diagnosed with squamous cell carcinoma of the lower lip. The youngest patient was 39 years old; the oldest patient was 76 years old. In this patient population, one patient had already been treated with radiation therapy 25 years ago after diagnosis of squamous cell carcinoma. The method was performed on four patients using bilateral flaps. On the other four patients, it was sufficient to use the advancement-rotation flap technique on one side.

时至今日，文中介绍的方法还无法被证实能够运用于全下唇缺失的重建修复。当时在我们的患者人群中，没有患者由于肿瘤需要进行下唇完全切除。理论上我们的新方法也可以和BERNARD–FRIES方法一样运用于全下唇替代。

To this day, this technique has not been implemented for reconstruction after full loss of the lower lip.

In our patient population in this period of time, there was no patient with a tumor that extensive that would have made a complete resection of the lower lip necessary. Generally, our method, as well as the technique by BERNARD-FRIES, is suitable for reconstruction of the entire lip.

术后定期进行肿瘤复查，至今无复发病例。再造的下唇功能基本上达到令人满意的程度。

Postoperatively, tumor control examinations were conducted at regular intervals. No recurrence was found to date. In general, the function of the reconstructed lower lip can be referred to as highly satisfactory.

接下来还必须对于手术技术的专门问题和所产生的结果进行深入的讨论：

Hereinafter, specific problems of the operative technique and consequences are discussed in detail:

1. 下唇再造后的瘢痕位于鼻唇沟与表情肌皮肤张力线区域。

1. Scarring after reconstruction of the lower lip should be located in the area of the nasolabial fold and the mimic skin tension lines.

通过观察，鼻唇沟从鼻翼成30° 角向尾部延伸至两侧嘴角区域。在此与位于两侧嘴角1.5cm点处垂直向下的嘴角皱纹融合。鼻唇沟与嘴角皱纹的深度对于别的面部皮肤纹路来说更取决于年龄。皮肤的弹性越差，这两条纹路就越深。重合于此皮肤张力线的瘢痕通常不明显。

According to our own observations, the nasolabial fold stretches from the wing of the nose in a 30° angle in caudal direction towards the lateral commissure of the mouth. It continues into the oral commissure fold, which, from this point, drags on vertically downwards from approximately 1.5 cm lateral of the oral commissure. Depending on age, the nasolabial and oral commissure folds are deeper than the remaining skin folds. The higher the loss of elasticity of the skin, the deeper the resulting folds. Scarring along these tension lines usually is less noticeable.

通过BERNARD方法再造的下唇，鼻唇沟瘢痕止于嘴角区域。

According to the reconstruction of the lower lip by BERNARD, the nasolabial scars end in the oral commissure area.

此外，由于运用此方法时，切除的Burrow氏三角牺牲了口周围组织，使得再造的下唇相对过窄。切除的Burrow氏三角，在鼻唇沟区域形成的瘢痕与鼻唇沟的走向不重合，从而在审美上达不到令人满意的效果。

Furthermore, using this method, the new lower lip seems to be too tight due to the loss of pe-rioral tissue as part of the excision of Burrow's triangles. Scarring after excision of these Burrow's triangles in the nasolabial area does not match the nasolabial fold lines and therefore does not allow for an aesthetically satisfactory result.

FRIES改进了BERNARD的手术。其中将Burrow氏三角的基部稍稍向上弯曲，从而使其与鼻唇沟相吻合。

FRIES modified the operation technique by BERNARD by making the base of the Burrow's triangles proceed upwards in a slightly curved direction to follow the nasolabial fold.

术后形成的向上弯曲的瘢痕可能影响手术的审美效果。

This upwardly curved scarring possibly compromises the aesthetic result postoperatively.

用GILLIES再造方法所形成的瘢痕超出鼻唇沟范围，从而特别明显。同时还会在唇基部由于组织隆起形成"猫耳"。

The reconstruction method according to GILLIES indicates initial scarring outside of the nasolabial fold and is thus exceptionally noticeable. Additionally, a formation of raised tissue rims on the base of the flap can be observed, also known as "dog-ear or pig-ear".

采用McGREGOR方法，皮肤的隆起状况较小，口裂相对较大。

These skin duplicates become smaller and the oral fissure relatively larger when using the method by McGREGOR.

NAKAJIMA等描述了另一种方法。此方法将皮瓣蒂部形成于面动脉而不是唇动脉。由此使切口靠近上唇红边缘，从而避免"猫耳"的形成。这种方法的缺点也是术后形成的瘢痕不与鼻唇沟重合。

NAKAJIMA et al. presented an alternative. Using their reconstruction method, the pedicle of the flap is not formed at the arteria labialis but at the arteria facialis. This allows for an incision all the way to the edge of the upper lip vermilion and by that prevents the development of "dog-ear or pig-ear". A disadvantage of this method is scarring that does not follow the nasolabial fold line.

本文中介绍的下唇再造方法，术后形成的瘢痕与实际鼻唇沟重合，从而实现审美与功能上令人满意的效果。

The method described here allows for a reconstruction of the lower lip in which the subsequent scar line accurately follows the nasolabial fold and therefore guarantees an aesthetically as well as functionally satisfying result.

2. 下唇再造的目的是重建一个两边对称的下唇。如果癌肿的位置居正中或旁正中，缺损通常采用推进皮瓣或旋转皮瓣来修补。

2. The reconstruction of the lower lip aims for a bilateral symmetry of the lower lip. If the carcinoma is situated in the center or paramedian of the lower lip, most defect coverage is performed using advancement or rotation flaps.

对于两侧皮瓣修复多数会形成对称的瘢痕。

If the formation of flaps is bilateral, a symmetric scarring is the result in the majority of cases.

运用本文介绍的自创下唇再造方法，对于两侧皮瓣使用可获得对称的下唇。根据我的经验，对于单侧使用旋转-推进复合皮瓣的情况，可获得比使用FRIES和GILLIES方法更对称的下唇。

The reconstruction of the lower lip with the method outlined above will allow for symmetric lower lips when performed bilaterally. According to my own experience, even a unilateral execution of the combined rotation-advancement flap is more likely to provide for a more symmetrical lower lip than the technique by FRIES and GILLIES could offer.

在运用BERNARD-FRIES方法再造下唇后显示手术侧明显比健康一侧要紧张。

After performing a reconstruction using the BERNARD-FRIES technique, the operated side seems considerably tenser than the healthy side.

在根据GILLES方法使用扇形皮瓣后，手术侧嘴角高度要高于对侧嘴角而且结构更多地呈椭圆形。这一特点导致了嘴部非对称的印象。

After unilateral application of the GILLIES fan flap, the oral commissure of the operated side is higher than the contralateral oral commissure and is rather oval in its configuration. This gives the impression of an asymmetric mouth.

在运用McGREGOR方法后，这一不对称特点在张嘴状态下才显现。

Using the McGREGOR technique, this asymmetry is only visible when the mouth is opened.

另一个下唇再造修复的目的是理想的口裂宽度。在GILLIES方法中，下唇红由上唇唇红黏膜构成。这一方式的后果就使口裂变小且由于皮瓣置换使得两侧上唇区域向两侧尾部平移。由此需要二次手术来扩展口裂。

A further goal of the reconstruction of the lower lip is a sufficiently wide oral fissure. Following the GILLIES method, the lower lip vermilion is being reconstructed by using mucosa from the upper lip vermilion. This implicates that the oral fissure is scaled down and that a lateral and cranial shift of the lateral upper lip region results from the replacement flap. An expansion of the oral fissure has to be performed in a second operation.

我的经验也显示，采用此种方法也能获得一个对称的、足够宽度的口裂。

However, my own experiences have shown that using this technique also allows for a sufficiently wide oral fissure.

3. 相对于BERNARD方法或者FRIES方法，其经常被发现口裂扩大的结果，采用上面所介绍的新方法，口裂的宽度保持正常。

3. Following the new method outlined above, the size of rima oris does not change, contrary to the BERNARD or FRIES procedure where an enlargement of the oral fissure is observed frequently.

4. 下唇再造的另一个目的是避免术后的再造下唇的皮肤与原来有明显色差。

4. A further aim of lower lip reconstruction is to prevent color differences of the reconstructed skin compared to the original skin of the lip.

采用上述所介绍的近95种方法进行下唇再造，主要运用推进皮瓣和旋转皮瓣来完成，基本上可以完成所有因下唇肿瘤切除后的下唇缺损的修复。由于使用了邻近皮瓣，几乎没有色差。相反，由于非邻近皮瓣技术（管状皮瓣或双蒂肌黏膜瓣）修复区域与脸部皮肤总存在色差，肤色和皮肤纹理会显得不自然。

With regard to the 95 methods of lower lip reconstruction outlined in the body of this thesis that are mainly performed by formation of advancement and rotation flaps, generally all lower lip defects can be reconstructed after tumor excision. As these methods use local flaps, differences in color are unlikely to occur. On the contrary, the skin complexion after application of a distant flap grafting technique (tubed pedicle flap or bridge flap) will never match the facial skin. Both complexion and texture of the skin appear to be unnatural.

该文所介绍的新方法（即第96种）允许修复下唇时直接采用口周围组织，从而避免出现了肤色的差别。

The presented 96th method allows for reconstruction of the lower lip using tissue from the immediate vicinity of the mouth. Therefore, differences in color will not occur.

5. 下唇再造还有一个目的是尽可能地完整再造下唇的原始结构。这一目的决定了修复所采用的最好材料就是直接来源于缺损周围区域。与之相反，来自远端皮瓣组织的弹性与下唇区域的组织完全没有可比性。

5. Another objective of the reconstructed lower lip is the complete recreation of the original structure of the lower lip. Therefore, the most suitable reconstruction tissue originates from the immediate vicinity of the defect. On the contrary, the elasticity of the tissue of a distant flap can not be compared to the tissue of the lower lip area.

本文所介绍的新技术采用直接来自下唇区域的推进–旋转皮瓣，从而可取得相对于其他方法更理想的修复结果。

The method presented here uses advancement-rotation flaps from the immediate vicinity of the lower lip and therefore allows for a relatively ideal reconstruction result.

6. 另外，再造的下唇厚度与原先的下唇大小需相符。

6. Furthermore, the thickness of the reconstructed lip should be consistent with the original dimension of the lower lip.

运用GILLIES，BERNARD和FRIES方法再造下唇，结果与原来的下唇比较几乎没有可见的差别，但通常导致嘴角的偏移。

The techniques by GILLIES, BERNARD and FRIES allow for a reconstruction of the lower lip that does not show noticeable differences in thickness compared to the original, but will result in a relocation of the oral commissures on a regular basis.

运用McGREGOR方法修复的下唇不仅口角看起来增厚肥大，而且整个下唇也增厚肥大。原因是由于采用了丰满的面颊皮瓣。本文所介绍的方法由于实际上通过旋转部分皮瓣而不带肌肉组织，结果可以获得相比采用BERNARD，GILLIES或McGREGOR方法更具漂亮外形的口角区域。

Following the McGREGOR technique, not only the oral commissure but also the entire lower lip appears to be thickened and hypertrophic due to the utilization of the voluminous buccal flaps. The method mentioned here offers a more delicate formation of the oral commissure area compared to the techniques by BERNARD, GILLIES or McGREGOR due to the fact that a flap without muscle tissue is transposed.

7. 再造后的下唇应当不窄也不紧张，采用双侧GILLIES氏扇形皮瓣方法再造的下唇结果相对较小，但两边对称。运用McGREGOR方法通过90°旋转面颊皮瓣修复的下唇宽度足够，但由于选用的面颊皮瓣厚度，使得再造后的下唇过于肥厚。这一缺点对于单侧面颊皮瓣旋转尤其明显。

7. After reconstructing the lower lip, it should not be too narrow and tight. The bilateral GIL-LIES fan technique allows for a relatively small yet symmetric lower lip. Following the

McGREGOR procedure, a buccal flap is rotated 90° and results in a lower lip that has an ade-quate width but appears to be too voluminous due to the application of thick buccal flaps. This is particularly noticeable when performing a unilateral rotation of the buccal flap.

运用BERNARD-FRIES方法再造下唇，虽然可获得宽度足够的口裂，但同时由于口周区域组织紧张使得前庭变小。

The BERNARD-FRIES method results in a sufficiently wide oral fissure but a constricted oral vestibule and, at the same time, tense tissue in the perioral area.

本文所介绍的下唇再造方法避免了这种在下唇区域的紧张。手术后由于从下面颊推进皮瓣所形成的二次缺损将通过鼻唇沟区域的旋转皮瓣来修复，这就使得新形成的下唇的紧张程度减至最小。

The lower lip reconstruction method outlined above avoids this tension in the lower lip area. The secondary defect after reconstruction of the lower lip by advancement flap from the lower buccal area will be smoothed out by a rotation flap from the nasolabial area. This reduces the tension of the newly formed lower lip.

8. 下唇再造的主要目的还在于重视口裂的功能。基于嘴唇的活动性的考虑，自然是邻位，邻近皮瓣要大大优于远位皮瓣。

8. Primary goal of the reconstruction of the lower lip is the consideration of the function of the oral fissure. Considering the mobility of the lips, local flaps of all shapes are superior to distant flaps.

远位皮瓣再造下唇仅仅可用于修复缺损部位，术后无运动功能的情况，唇只能完全以被动方式运动。只要邻近皮瓣包含有口轮匝肌部分，则运用邻近皮瓣修复的方法所获得的活动状态要明显优于用其他方法。

Distant flaps serve solely for coverage of defects without providing mobility afterwards. Movement of the lips is only possible passively. If parts of orbicularis oris are preserved in a local flap, the mobility patterns are superior to alternative methods.

采用GILLIES方法修复下唇缺损时，虽然扇形皮瓣带有部分口轮匝肌，但在切割皮瓣时，切到了上唇提肌部分、颧大肌部分、笑肌部分、降口角肌部分以及下唇降肌部分。由于这一原因使再造的唇部的运动功能必然受到损害。同时由于切断了感觉神经，从而使其丧失部分敏感度。在根据McGREGOR对于此扇形皮瓣的改进中同样损伤到了感觉和运动神经分布。对于面部神经的损伤所造成的功能障碍要大于口轮匝肌受损所造成的后果。

According to the GILLIES method the fan flap includes parts of orbicularis oris; however, when completely dissecting the flap, parts of levator labii superioris, zygomaticus majoris, risorius, depressor anguli oris as well as depressor labii inferioris are cut through. Therefore, the mobility of the reconstructed lip will be impaired. Additionally, transection of sensory nerve branches simultaneously results in a loss of sensibility. The modified McGREGOR fan flap also leads to damage of sensory and motor innervation. A damage of the facial branches involves a more significant dysfunction compared to the full separation of orbicularis oris.

将BERNARD技术与根据FRIES改良的方法做比较，发现FRIES方法要优于BERNARD技术，因为前者无须切割到口轮匝肌。

Comparing the BERNARD technique with the FRIES modification, the FRIES method is superior to the technique by BERNARD as it does not require the excision of parts of orbicularis oris.

当采用FRIES技术时，口轮匝肌将被切开。但同时仍然切断了环状肌的连续性，这导致表情非常僵硬。

Following the FRIES technique, the orbicularis oris muscle is merely cut through. However, the continuity of the orbicularis muscle is interrupted, which leads to a certain rigid mimic expression.

采用本文介绍的新方法，在口角区域内侧部切开时可最少保留一半口轮匝肌，从而保证了部分口轮匝肌的连续性。拆线后唇部的灵活性就已经证明了口轮匝肌的连续性。因为取自鼻唇沟区域的旋转皮瓣主要包含皮肤，或者对于大型下唇缺损主要是皮肤以及部分肌肉，其不会对上唇肌肉的功能造成损害。由于取自鼻唇沟区域的旋转皮瓣大小有限，手术部位的感觉神经支配的恢复也加快。

With the new method outlined above, at least half of orbicularis oris is preserved while the medial part is cut through in the commissure of the mouth. This way, the continuity of orbicularis oris is kept intact at least partially. After suture removal, the excellent mobility of the lips proves the continuity of orbicularis oris. As rotation flaps of the nasolabial area mainly contain skin, or skin and muscle tissue in larger lower lip defects, the function of the upper lip muscles is not impaired. Due to the limited size of rotation flaps taken from the nasolabial area, the sensory reinnervation of the surgical area progresses rapidly.

9. 下唇再造术另一个优点是方法的一次性。

9. Another advantage of lower lip reconstruction is the simultaneousness of a method.

运用远位皮瓣理所当然需要多个手术步骤。这会对患者造成心理上的负担，同时由于长时间的住院而产生高昂的费用。出于该原因，采用邻近皮瓣有所禁忌或不可能时，远位皮瓣修复术才考虑采用。

Distant flaps naturally require several operation steps. This leads to psychological stress for the patient and higher cost due to additional hospital stays. For this reason, distant flap techniques will be reserved for such situations wherein any local flap method is either contraindicated or impossible.

同样采用邻近皮瓣重建术也不总是被考虑一次性手术，比如根据GILLIES方法重建要求进行二次手术来修正圆钝的嘴角。本文所介绍的方法同BERNARD方法和FRIES方法一样只做一次性手术。

However, the local flap reconstruction does not always allow for a single operation. For example, the GILLIES reconstruction method requires a second operation for the reconstruction of the rounded oral commissure. The method outlined here, as well as the BERNARD and FRIES technique, is only performed in a single session.

10. 当由于原有的疾病而麻醉风险高时，下唇再造手术也可在局部麻醉下进行。多数邻近皮瓣整形可在局部麻醉下一个步骤完成。

10. If there is a high anesthetic risk due to a preexisting condition, the lip reconstruction can also be performed under local anaesthesia. Most local flap techniques are suitable for operation under local anaesthesia.

本文介绍的方法由于向面颊区域扩张较小，且仅局限于口周范围，所以也可在局部麻醉下实施。在我们的患者中，局部麻醉下实施重建手术效果令人满意。

The method presented here allows for execution under local anaesthesia due to its limited expansion into the buccal and perioral area. In our patient population, the results of reconstruction under local anaesthesia were satisfactory.

11. 还有一个对于所采用的皮瓣可靠性重要的标准是其供血的血管蒂即皮瓣基部的宽度。

11. An additional essential criterion for the safety of a used flap is its afferent vascular pedicle or rather the width of its base.

大面积和大体积皮瓣经常被发现发生术后坏死。小皮瓣极少出现坏死的情况，同样当重要的血管如唇动脉受到损伤时也很少出现坏死。原因是可通过黏膜或渗透获取营养。

Postoperative necroses are more often observed in expanded and voluminous flaps. Due to nourishment from mucosa or by diffusion, smaller flaps show necrosis less often even if a dominant vessel, e.g. arteria labialis, is damaged.

根据整形外科任意皮瓣长宽比的基本原则，要求长宽比为2∶1，这在面部整形上不适用。由于丰富的血液供应，形成任意皮瓣长宽比可达3∶1到4∶1。如果此类皮瓣带有上唇动脉，则可视之为动脉化皮瓣，从而允许其长宽比甚至更大。

The ground rules of length-to-width ratio of randomized flaps in plastic surgery that require a length-to-width ratio of 2∶1 on the trunk, do not apply for the face. Due to the extraordinarily abundant blood supply, the creation of randomized flaps with a length-to-width ratio of 3∶1 to 4∶1 is possible. If such a flap contains the labialis superior arteria, it can be viewed as arterialized. By this, an even larger length-to-width ratio is tolerated.

BERNARD和FRIES方法中皮瓣蒂部非常宽。因此皮瓣的供血不会被破坏。本文所介绍的方法同样不会损伤推进皮瓣和旋转皮瓣的供血。良好的供血可以避免感染和感染引发的创面坏死。

According to the BERNARD and FRIES technique, there are exceedingly wide flap pedicles. Therefore, the blood supply is not impaired. In not one case did the method outlined here compromise the blood supply of the advancement or rotation flaps. Additionally, the good blood supply prevented infections and infection-induced necroses of wounds.

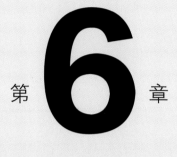

第**6**章

Chapter 6

总结

Summary

参考文献有记载以来，运用外科技术再造下唇缺损已有近200年。本文论述了95种不同的下唇再造的方法。连同我的手术方法共96种，这些方法主要分为3种方式：直接缝合、邻近皮瓣以及远位皮瓣。

Surgical techniques for the reconstruction of lower lip defects have been described in literature for nearly 200 years. In this thesis, 95 different methods for reconstruction of the lower lip are described. There are together 96 Methods with my own operative Technique. Primarily, three different types of reconstruction methods are differentiated: direct approximation, local flap as well as distant flap diagnostics.

在本文中对于邻近皮瓣技术进行了详细的鉴别和比较。

In this thesis, local flap methods are presented in detail.

其主要分为两种类型：推进皮瓣（例如BERNARD方法）；旋转皮瓣（例如GILLIES方法）。

Two types are differentiated in regard to those methods: The advancement flap (e.g. the BERNARD technique); The rotation flap (e.g. the GILLIES technique).

此外还介绍了一种全新的肌功能的方法来实施下唇缺损后的修复重建。该技术由一推进皮瓣和一旋转皮瓣组合形成。此外，该技术还避免了运用BERNARD-FRIES方法所需要的Burrow氏三角的切除。由于避免了舍弃非病变肌肉皮肤区域，使得采用本书描述的新方法可形成完全对称作用的唇，同样也可避免由于组织凸起形成的"猫耳"。

Furthermore, a new myofunctional method for reconstruction after lower lip defects is presented. This technique consists of a combination of an advancement and rotation flap. In addition, the technique avoids the excision of Burrow's triangles which are used in the BERNARD-FRIES technique. Avoiding distortions of healthy myocutaneous areas with the method outlined here, allows for the creation of a lip that appears to be symmetrical. Raised tissue known as "dog-ear or pig-ear" can be avoided as well.

与其他再造技术方法相比较，迄今为止在8位患者身上获得的经验显示出了功能和审美上的非常良好的效果。

Our past experience with eight patients showed a very good functional and aesthetic result compared to alternative reconstruction methods.

肌功能推进-旋转皮瓣整形有如下优点：

（1）下唇修复后形成的瘢痕位于鼻唇沟区域和口周区的微小皮肤张力线里。

（2）该方法可再造出对称的下唇。

（3）术后口裂宽度与术前对应一致。

（4）由于应用邻近皮瓣，术后不会出现色差。

（5）由于在口角区域仅局部切断口轮匝肌，再造的厚度与术前下唇厚度一致。无凸起和张力。

（6）由于局部保留口轮匝肌，术后1周就表现出功能上的良好效果。

（7）当全麻风险高时，此方法可以在局部麻醉下进行。

（8）该技术可单侧，也可双侧进行，所应用的皮瓣蒂部宽度不影响推进皮瓣及旋转皮瓣的活力。

The advantages of myofunctional advancement-rotation flaps are as follows:

（1）Scarring after reconstruction of the lower lip is located in the nasolabial fold and the minimal skin tension lines of the perioral area.

（2）This method allows for the creation of a symmetrical lower lip.

（3）The width of the reconstructed oral fissure is equivalent to the preoperative situation.

（4）Due to application of local flaps, there are no postoperative differences in color.

（5）Due to the solely partial cut of the orbicularis oris muscle in the oral commissure area, the thickness of the reconstruction result is equivalent to the preoperative dimension of the lower lip. Raised tissue and tensile strains do not occur.

（6）Due to partial preservation of orbicularis oris, a good functional result was achieved as early as one week postoperatively.

（7）This method can be carried out under local anaesthesia in case of anesthetic risk.

（8）The technique can be performed unilaterally as well as bilaterally, the width of the used base of the flap does not lead to exposed vitality of advancement or rotation flaps.

7

第 章

Chapter 7

参考文献

Reference

[1] ABBE R. A new plastic operation for the relief of deformity due to double hare lip[J]. Med. Rec., 1898, 53: 477.

[2] ANDREWS E B. Repair of lower lip defects by the Hagedorn rectangular flap method[J]. Plastic and Reconstructive Surgery, 1964, 34: 27.

[3] ASHLEY F L. Reconstruction of the lower lip[J]. Plastic and Reconstructive Surgery, 1955, 15: 313.

[4] BAKAMJIAN V. Use of tongue flaps in lower lip reconstruction[J]. British Journal of Plastic Surgery, 1964, 17: 76.

[5] BARTON M, SPIRA M, HARDY S B. An improved method for "V" excision of the lip combined with vermilionectomy[J]. Plastic and Reconstructive Surgery, 1964, 33: 471.

[6] BERNARD C. Cancer de la levre inferieure restauration a l'aide de lam-beaux quadrilaterires-lateraux querison[J]. Scalpel. Liege, 1851, 5: 162.

[7] BRETTEVILLE-JENSEN G. Reconstruction of the lower lip after central excision[J]. British Journal of Plastic Surgery, 1973, 26: 247.

[8] BROMLEY S. Myoplastic Modification of the Bernard Cheiloplasty[J].Plastic and Reconstructive Surgery, 1958, 21: 453.

[9]BROADBENT T R, MATHEWS V I.Artistic Relationships in Surface Anatomy of the face. Application to Reconstructive Surgery[J]. Plastic and Reconstructive Surgery,1957, 20: 2.

[10]BRUNS V. Chirurgische Mitteilungen[J]. Archiv für Physiologische Heilkunde, 1844, 31: 34.

[11]BRUNS V. Handbuch der praktischen Chirurgie[M]. Tübingen: Laup, 1859.

[12]BUROW C A. Beschreibung einer neuen Transplantations-Methode (Methode der seitlichen Dreiecke) zum Wiederersatz verlorengegangener Teile des Gesichts[M]. Berlin: Nauck, 1855.

[13]CONLEY J. Malignant tumours of the scalp[J]. Plastic and Reconstructive Surg, 1964, 33: 1.

[14]CONVERSE, J M. WOOD-SMITH, D.Techniques for the repair of defects of the lips and cheeks[J]. Reconstructive Plastic Surgery, 1977, 3: 1544.

[15]DAVIS J S.Plastic Surgery, Its Principles and Practice[M]. Philadelphia: Blakiston, 1919: 543.

[16]DIEFFENBACH J F. Chirurgische Erfahrungen[M]. 101 Berlin: Berlin, 1834.

[17]ESSERN J F S.Gestielte lokale Nasenplastik mit zweizipfligen Lappen, Deckung des sekundären Defektes vom ersten Zipfel durch den zweiten[J]. Deutsche Zeitschrift für Chir., 1918, 143: 385.

[18]ESTLANDER J A. Classic Reprint: A method of reconstructing loss of substance in one lip from the other lip Arch[J]. Klin. Chir., 1872, 14: 622.

[19]FERNER H. Atlas der topographischen und angewandten Anatomie des Menschen[M]. München-Wien-Baltimor: Urban & Schwarzenberg, 1980.

[20]FREEMAN B S. Myoplastic modification of the Bernard cheiloplasty[J]. Plastic and Reconstructive Surg, 1958, 21: 453.

[21]FRIES R. Über eine neue Methode der primären Wiederherstellung des Mundwinkels nach Carcinom-exstirpation[J]. Österr. Z. Stomat, 1962, 59: 366.

[22]FRIES R. Vorzug der Bernardschen Operation als Universalverfah-ren zur Rekonstruktion der Unterlippe. Carcinomresektion. Chir. Plastica[M]. Berlin: Springer verlag, 1971.

[23]FRIES R. Advantages of a Basic Concept in Lip Reconstruction after Tumour Resection[J]. J max.-fac. Surg, 1973, 1: 13.

[24]FUJIMORI R, HIRAMOTO M. OFUJI S.Sponge fixation method for the treatment of early scars[J]. Plastic and Reconstructive Surg, 1968, 42: 322.

[25]FUJIMORI R. Gate flap for total reconstruction of lower lip. Brit[J]. Journal of Plastic Surg. 1980, 33: 345.

[26]GILLIES H D, MILLARD D R.Principles and Art of Plastic Surgery[M]. Boston: Little, Brown & Co., 1957.

[27]GOLDSTEIN M H. A Tissue-Expanding Vermilion Myocutaneous Flap for Lip Repair[J]. Plastic and Reconstructive Surg,1984, 73: 768.

[28]GOLDSTEIN M H. Orbiting the orbicularis: Restoration of muscle-ring continuity with myocutaneous flaps[J]. Plastic and Reconstructive Surg. 1983, 72: 294.

[29]GORM BRETTERVILLE-JENSEN. Reconstruction of the lower lip after central excisions[J]. P. R. S, 1973, 26: 247.

[30]GRIMM G. Eine neue Methode der Nahlappenplastik zum Ersatz tumorbedingter totaler Unterlippendefekte[J]. Zentralbl. Chir., 1966, 91: 1621.

[31]GÜNTHER H. SPIESSL B.Rekonstruktion der Unterlippe nach Carcinomentfernung und gleichzeitiger Ausräumung regionärer Lymphknoten[J]. Chir. Plast. Reconstr, 1967, 3: 230.

[32]GÜNTHER H. Die chirurgische Behandlung des Unterlippencarcinoms[J]. Fortschr. Kiefer- u. Gesichtschir, 1968, 13: 118.

[33]GÜNTHER H. Lippenschleimhautersatz im Rahmen der Rekonstruktion der Unterlippe[J]. Dtsch. Zahn-, Mund- u. Kieferheilk, 1966, 47: 321.

[34]HOLMSTRAND K, LONGACRE J J. STEFANO, G.The ultrastructure of collagen in skin, scards and keloids[J]. Plastic and Reconstructive Surg, 1961, 27: 597.

[35]JABALEY M E, CLEMENT R L, ORGUTT T W. Myocutaneous flaps in lip reconstruction (applications of the Karapandzic principle)[J]. P.R.S., 1977, 59: 680.

[36]JAMES S, MYERS EN. Cancer of the Head and Neck[M]. New York: Churchill Livingstone, 1981.

[37]JOHANSON B. ASPELUND E. BREIN U. HOMSTROM, H.Surgical treatment of non-traumatic lower lip lesions with special reference to the step technique (a follow up 149 patients)[J]. Scand. J. Plast. Reconstr. Surg, 1974, 8: 232.

[38]KARAPANDZIC M. Reconstruction of lip defects by local arterial flaps[J]. Brit. J. Plast. Surg, 1974, 27: 93.

[39]LE MESURIER A B. A method of cutting and suturing the lip in the treatment of complete unilateral clefts[J]. Plastic and Reconstructive Surg,1949, 4: 1.

[40]LENTRODT J, LUHR H G. Reconstruction of the lower lip after tumour resection combined with radical neck dissection[J]. Plastic and Reconstructive Surg, 1971, 48: 579.

[41]LONGENECKER C G, RYAN R F.Cancer of the lip in a large charity hospital[J]. Southern Medical Journal, 1965, 58: 1459.

[42]MARTIN H E. Cheiloplasty for advanced carcinoma of the lip[J]. Surg. Gynec. and Obst, 1932, 54: 914.

[43]MAY H. One-Stage operation for closure of large defects of the lower lip and chin[J]. Surg. Gynec. and Obst, 1941, 73: 236.

[44]MAY H. Closure of defects of lips with composite vermilion bor-der-lined flaps[J]. Ann. Surg,1944, 120: 241.

[45]MAY H. The modified Dieffenbach operation for closure of large defects of the lower lip and chin[J]. Plastic and Reconstructive Surg, 1946, 1: 194.

[46]MAY H. Reconstruction and Reparative Surgery[M]. Philadelphia: F.A. Davis Company, 1947.

[47]MAY H. Surgical treatment of carcinoma of the lip[J]. Plastic and Reconstructive Surg, 1952, 9: 424.

[48]McGREGOR I A. The tongue flap in lip surgery[J]. Brit. Journ. of Plastic Surg, 1966, 19: 253.

[49]McGREGOR I A. Reconstruction of the lower lip[J]. Brit. Journ. Plast. Surg, 1983, 36: 40.

[50]MEYER W. Die Zahn-, Mund- und Kieferheilkunde[M]. 2nd ed. Berlin: Urban & Schwarzenberg, 1955.

[51]MÖRIKE K D. Lehrbuch der makroskopischen Anatomie für Zahnärzte[M]. Stuttgart: Gustav Fischer, 1969.

[52]NAKAJIMA T, YOSHIMURA T, KAMI T. Reconstruction of the lower lip with a fan-shaped flap based on the facial artery[J]. Brit. Journ. Plast. Surg, 1984, 37: 52.

[53]NAUMANN H H. Kopf- und Hals-Chirurgie[M]. Stattgart: Thieme, 1974.

[54]NELATON C. OMBREDANNE L. Les Autoplastics Leures, Joues, Orsille, Tronc, Membres[M]. Paris: G. Steinheil, 1907.

[55]NEW G B. The repair of post-operative defects involving the lips and cheeks secondary to the removal of malignant tumors[J]. Surg. Gynec. and Obst, 1936, 62: 182.

[56]PERON J M, ANDRIEU-GUITRANCOURT J, DEHESDIN D, FURET A.Reconstructions des pertes de substance de la lèvre inféri-eure[J]. Rev. Stomatol. Chir. Maxillofac, 1984, 85: 4302.

[57]RAVDIN I S. Kirschner's Operative Surgery English Translation[J]. J.B. Lippincott Co., 1931: 378.

[58]REHRMANN A. Rekonstruktion der Lippen nach Tumorentfernung[J]. Organ der Deutschen Gesellschaft für Plastische und Wiederherstellungs-Chirurgie, 1967, Bd. 3: 222.

[59]ROHEN J W. Funktionelle Anatomie des Menschen[M]. Stuttgard: Schattauer, 1973.

[60]ROHEN J W, YOKOCHI C. Anatomie des Menschen[M]. Stuttgart-New York: Schattauer, 1982.

[61]RUBIN L R. Langer's lines and facial scards[J]. Plastic and Reconstructive Surg, 1948, 3: 147.

[62]SCHUCHARDT K. Der Rundstiellappen in der Wiederherstellungschirurgie des Gesichts-Kieferbereichs[M]. Leipzig: Thieme, 1944.

[63]SCHUCHARDT K. Fortschr D. Kiefer- u. Gesichtschir[M]. Stuttgard: Thieme, 1966, 11: 27.

[64]SCHUCHARDT K. Grundsätzliches zur primären und sekundären Defektdeckung nach der Operation von gutartigen und bösartigen Gesichtstumoren[J]. Chir. Plast. Reconstruct, 1967, 5: 180.

[65]SMITH F. Some refinements in reconstructive surgery of the face[J]. J. Amer. Med. Ass, 1942, 120: 352.

[66]SPIESSL B. Möglichkeiten der Schnittführung zur en-bloc Resektion von fortgeschrittenen regionär metastasierenden Tumoren der Mundhöhle und des Gesichtes[J]. Dtsch. Zahn-, Mund- u. Kieferheilk, 1964, 43: 190.

[67]SPIRA M, HARDY S B. Vermilionectomy[J]. Plastic and Reconstructive Surg, 1964, 33: 39.

[68]STRANG M F, ROBERTSON G A. Steeple flap reconstruction of the lower lip[J]. Ann. Plast. Surg, 1983, 10: 4.

[69]STRANG M F, PAGE R E. Functional aspects of the reconstructed lip[J]. Ann. Plast. Surg, 1983, 10: 103.

[70]TÖNDURY G. Angewandte and topographische Anatomie[M]. Stuttgant: Thieme, 1959.

[71]ULLIK R. Die plastische Chirurgie des Gesichtes[M]. Wien: Urban u. Schwarzenberg, 1948.

[72]WEBSTER R C, COFFEY R J. KELLEHER, R.E. Total and partial reconstruction of the lower lip with innervated muscle-bearing flaps[J]. Plastic and Reconstructive Surg, 1960, 25: 360.

[73]WEISMAN P A.Angioma in the lips: An unresolved problem[J]. Plast. Reconstruct. Surg, 1961, 28: 43.

[74]ZIMANY A. The bi-lobe flap[J]. Plastic and Reconstructive Surg,1953, 11: 424.